AF746013

Primary Intracranial Tumors

Edited by Erasmo Barros Da Silva Junior and Jerônimo Buzetti Milano

Published in London, United Kingdom

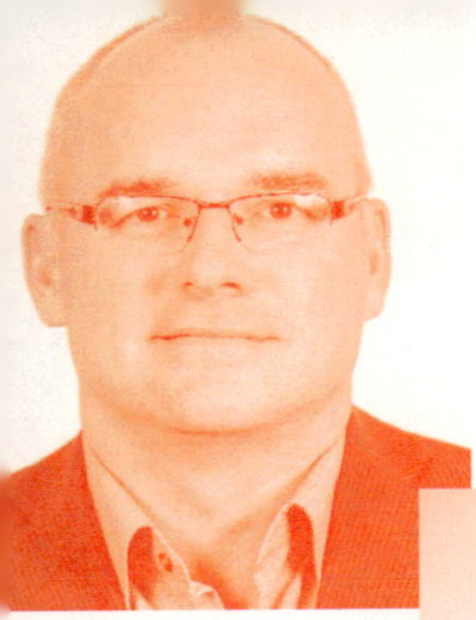
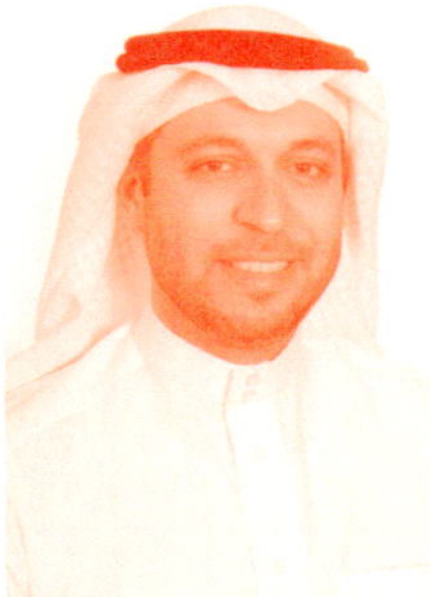
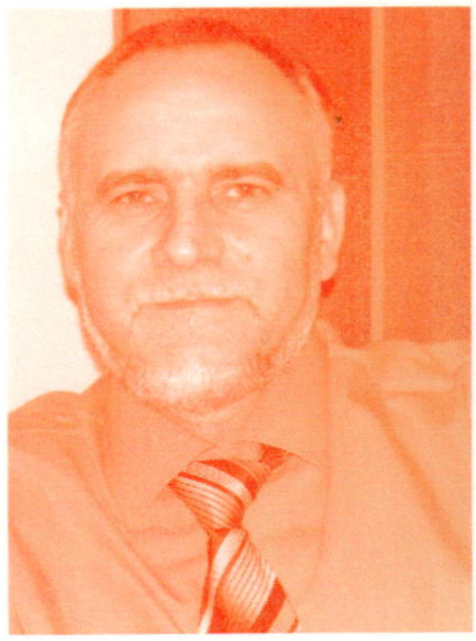
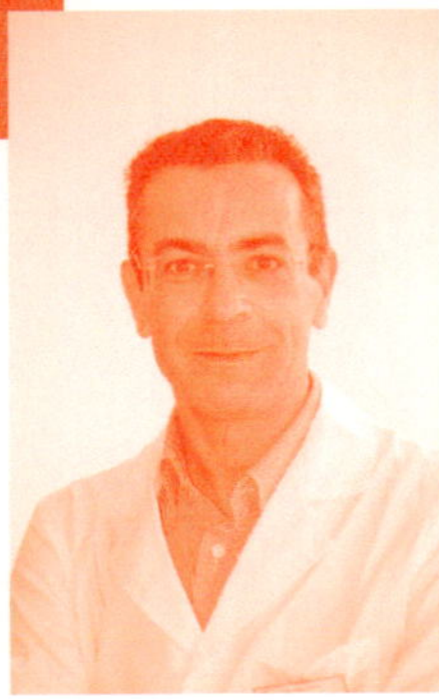
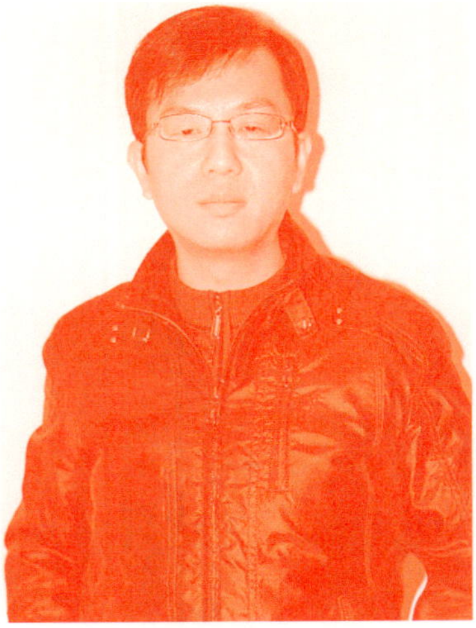
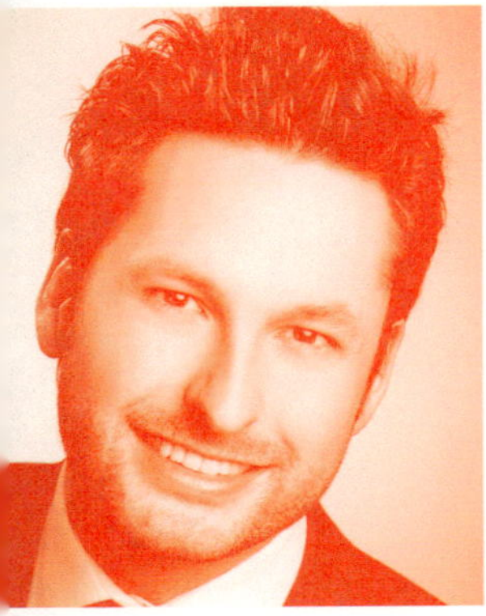
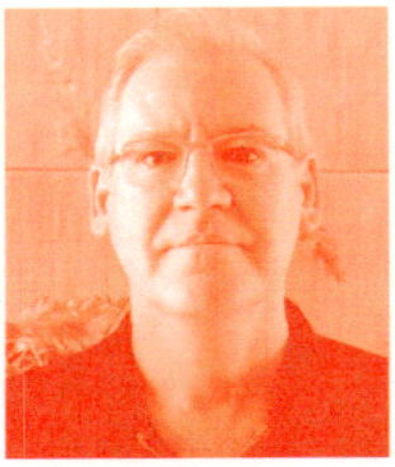

IntechOpen

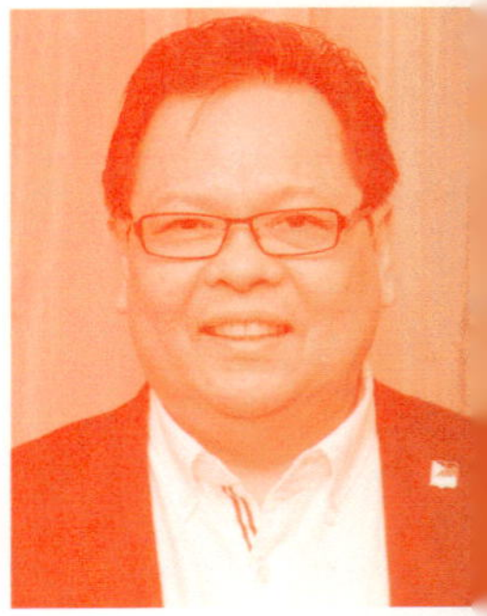
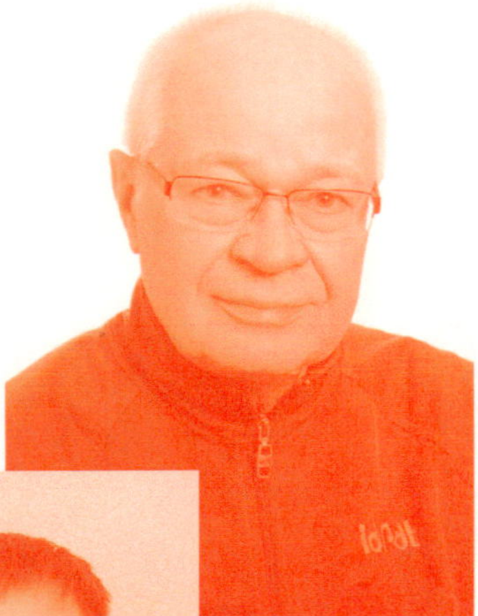
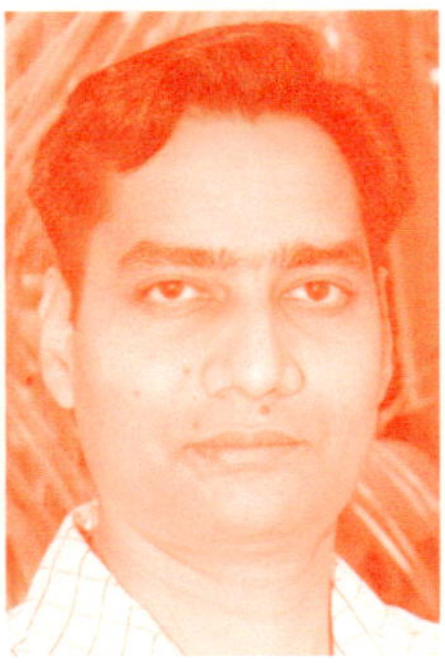
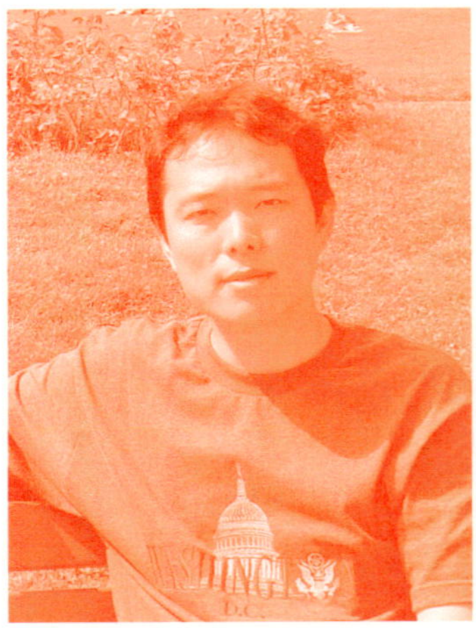
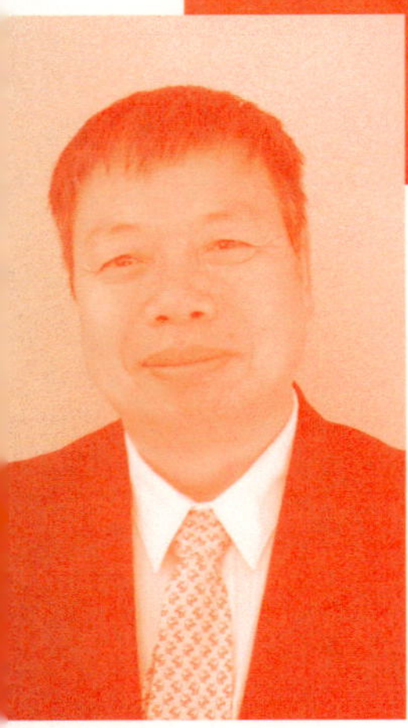
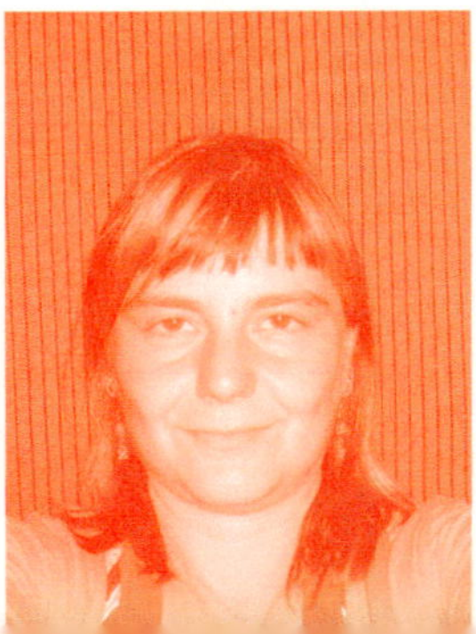

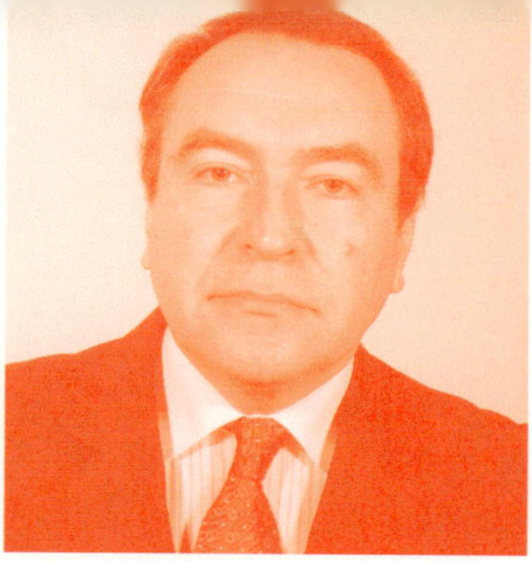
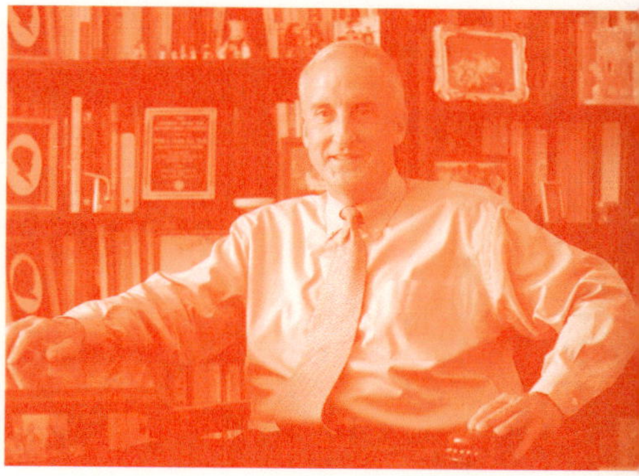
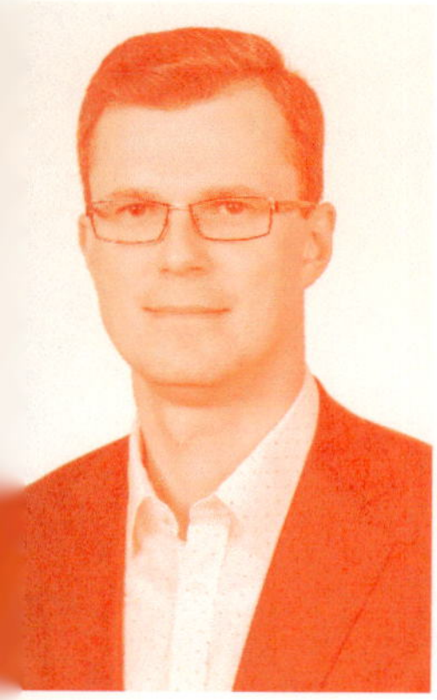
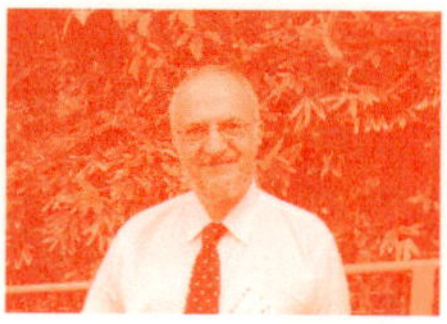
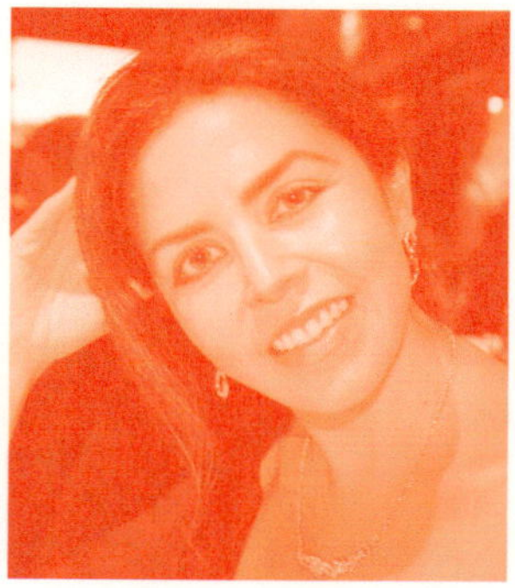

Supporting open minds since 2005

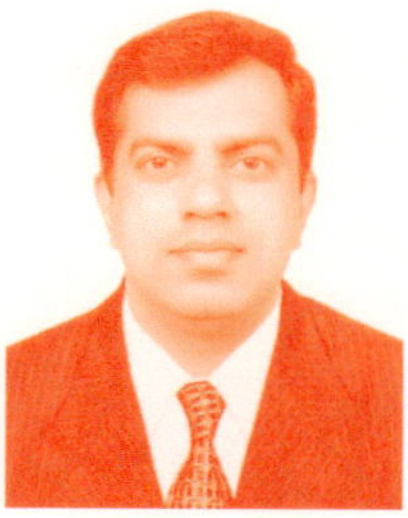
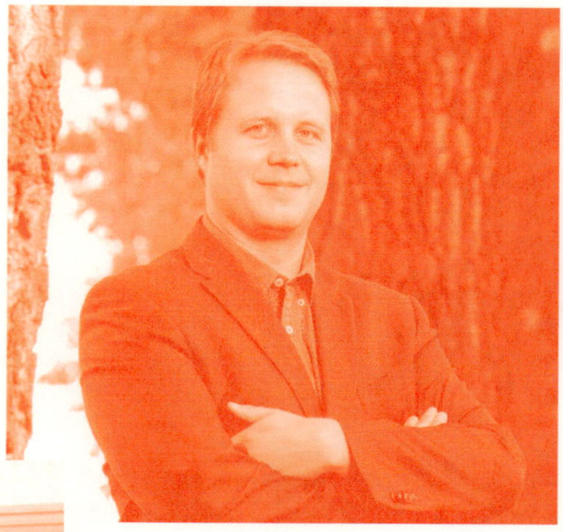
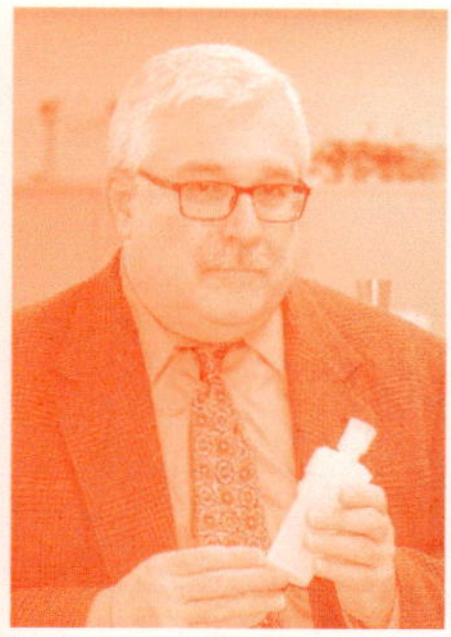
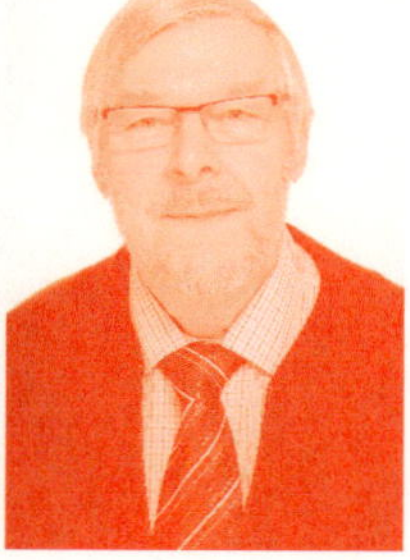
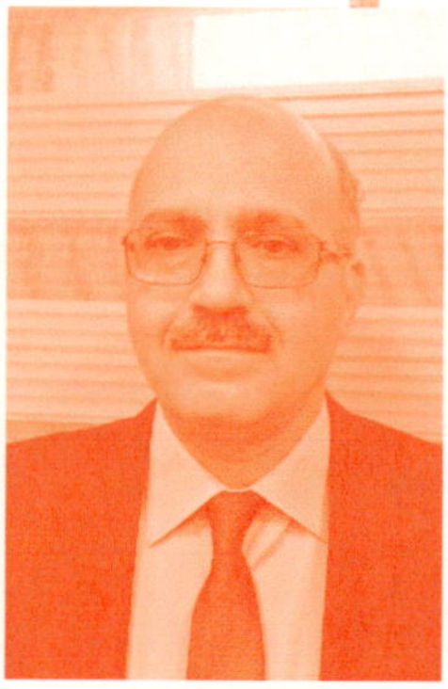
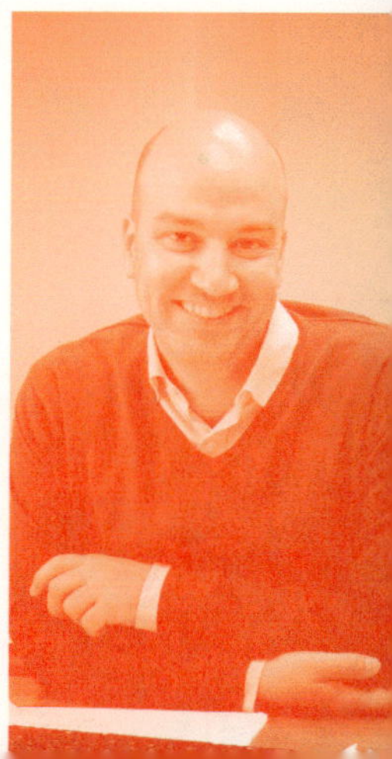
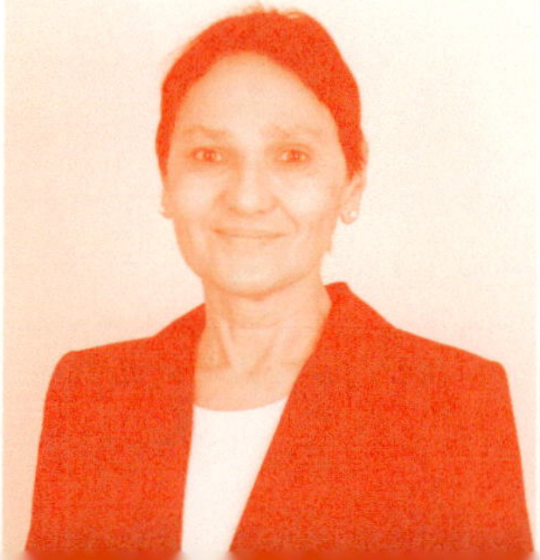

Primary Intracranial Tumors
http://dx.doi.org/10.5772/intechopen.75418
Edited by Erasmo Barros Da Silva Junior and Jerônimo Buzetti Milano

Contributors
Miguel Velázquez, Ruth Ruiz Esparza, Alicia Siordia, Griselda Ramírez, Gerardo Sánchez, Luis Fernando Moura Da Silva Jr., Henrique Balloni, Johnny Camargo, Gustavo Jung, Ricardo Ramina, Erasmo Barros Da Silva Junior, Joseph Franklin Chenisz Da Silva, Yuan Shan, Renzhi Wang

© The Editor(s) and the Author(s) 2019
The rights of the editor(s) and the author(s) have been asserted in accordance with the Copyright, Designs and Patents Act 1988. All rights to the book as a whole are reserved by INTECHOPEN LIMITED. The book as a whole (compilation) cannot be reproduced, distributed or used for commercial or non-commercial purposes without INTECHOPEN LIMITED's written permission. Enquiries concerning the use of the book should be directed to INTECHOPEN LIMITED rights and permissions department (permissions@intechopen.com).
Violations are liable to prosecution under the governing Copyright Law.

Individual chapters of this publication are distributed under the terms of the Creative Commons Attribution 3.0 Unported License which permits commercial use, distribution and reproduction of the individual chapters, provided the original author(s) and source publication are appropriately acknowledged. If so indicated, certain images may not be included under the Creative Commons license. In such cases users will need to obtain permission from the license holder to reproduce the material. More details and guidelines concerning content reuse and adaptation can be found at http://www.intechopen.com/copyright-policy.html.

Notice
Statements and opinions expressed in the chapters are these of the individual contributors and not necessarily those of the editors or publisher. No responsibility is accepted for the accuracy of information contained in the published chapters. The publisher assumes no responsibility for any damage or injury to persons or property arising out of the use of any materials, instructions, methods or ideas contained in the book.

First published in London, United Kingdom, 2019 by IntechOpen
IntechOpen is the global imprint of INTECHOPEN LIMITED, registered in England and Wales, registration number: 11086078, The Shard, 25th floor, 32 London Bridge Street
London, SE19SG – United Kingdom
Printed in Croatia

British Library Cataloguing-in-Publication Data
A catalogue record for this book is available from the British Library

Additional hard copies can be obtained from orders@intechopen.com

Primary Intracranial Tumors
Edited by Erasmo Barros Da Silva Junior and Jerônimo Buzetti Milano
p. cm.
Print ISBN 978-1-78985-405-3
Online ISBN 978-1-78985-406-0

For EU product safety concerns:
IN TECH d.o.o., Prolaz Marije Krucifikse Kozulić 3, 51000 Rijeka, Croatia, info@intechopen.com or visit our website at intechopen.com.

We are IntechOpen,
the world's leading publisher of
Open Access books
Built by scientists, for scientists

4,000+
Open access books available

116,000+
International authors and editors

120M+
Downloads

151
Countries delivered to

Our authors are among the
Top 1%
most cited scientists

12.2%
Contributors from top 500 universities

WEB OF SCIENCE™
Selection of our books indexed in the Book Citation Index
in Web of Science™ Core Collection (BKCI)

Interested in publishing with us?
Contact book.department@intechopen.com

Numbers displayed above are based on latest data collected.
For more information visit www.intechopen.com

Meet the editors

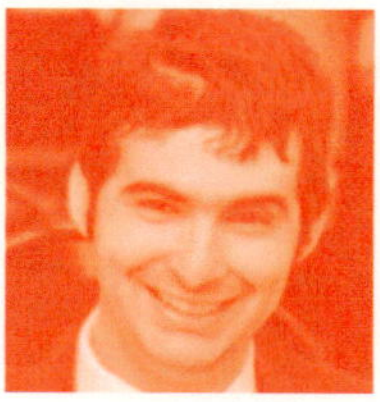

Erasmo Barros da Silva Junior is a specialist in neurosurgery at the Brazilian Society of Neurosurgery. He has a medical degree from the Federal University of Paraíba (2002) and a medical residency in neurosurgery at the Instituto de Neurologia de Curitiba (2004–2008). He has a Master's Degree in Surgery at PUC-PR (2007–2009). He is a titular member of the Brazilian Society of Neurosurgery and the Brazilian Academy of Neurosurgery, a member of the Society of Neuro-Oncology, a member of the European Association of Neurosurgical Societies (EANS), and a neurosurgeon at Instituto de Neurologia de Curitiba/Department of Neurosurgery/Neurooncology Division.

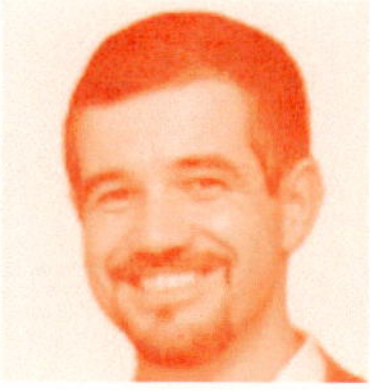

Jerônimo Buzetti Milano is a specialist in neurosurgery at the Brazilian Society of Neurosurgery. He has a medical degree from the Federal University of Paraná (2000) and a medical residency in neurosurgery at the Instituto de Neurologia de Curitiba (2001–2004). . He has a PhD in Neurology atUSP-SP (2006–2010). He is a titular member of the Brazilian Society of Neurosurgery and the Brazilian Academy of Neurosurgery, a member of Spine Brazilian Society, North American Spine Society, and AOSpine, a co-chair at the Fellowship in Neurosurgery of the World Federation of Neurosurgical Societies (WFNS), a professor at AOSpine Latin America, Postgraduation Course for Capacitation in Spine Surgery, and a neurosurgeon at Instituto de Neurologia de Curitiba/Department of Neurosurgery/Head, Spine Division.

Contents

Preface

Intracranial tumors represent a vast group of heterogeneous diseases, with complex and often challenging management, requiring specialized interdisciplinary teams in reference centers. Working with these professionals, focused on the most up-to-date behavior possible, is essential to alleviate patients' anxiety and discomfort.

The first successful removal of a brain tumor was described in 1879 by William Macewen. With the arrival of the 20th century, the foundations of modern neurosurgery were established by Cushing and incorporated the surgical microscope in intracranial operations, with House (in 1961 in acoustic tumors) and Kurze (in 1963), and improvements from Yasargil in the following decades. Also in the 1960s, dexamethasone was introduced in the treatment of tumor swelling and became one of the hallmarks for better patient survival.

In the 1970s, computed tomography and magnetic resonance imaging allowed intracranial structures to be visualized directly. Until then, tumors were diagnosed indirectly through invasive and dated examinations. They were delayed diagnoses and, invariably, patients presented with very severe conditions. At the same time, brain irradiation was incorporated in the treatment of malignant or unresectable tumors.

The 1980s and 1990s were decisive in the development of better imaging methods, surgical techniques, and estereotatic navigation for deep lesions. In the late 1990s, Stupp demonstrated the role of temozolamide in the treatment of glioblastomas, one of the most aggressive incurable cancers in humans. Improved monitoring conditions, neuroanesthesia, intensive care, and the increasing incorporation of technology in the service of medicine have made the management of brain tumors somewhat worthy of science fiction films. The current paradigms involve the application of tumor-treating fields, molecular analyses, biological markers, and advanced imaging techniques, all in continuous transformation, and trying to offer definitive solutions for the well-being of patients.

Such knowledge is like a regular polygon gaining more sides with each new discovery, trying to become a perfect "circle," although there are new questions that continuously arise the more we understand each disease. No matter how new divisions and classifications are created for a huge range of tumors, we can always improve the diagnostic methods, the surgery, and the adjuvant treatments.

This book presents specific and important topics about the most frequent primary intracranial tumors, highlighting the relevant contemporary literature and the experience of the services involved. They are fundamental information that, we hope, becomes out of date quickly, given the intensity with which one seeks to make the "polygon of knowledge" a "circle".

Erasmo Barros Da Silva Junior
Neurological Institute Of Curitiba, Brazil

Jerônimo Buzetti Milano
Neurological Institute Of Curitiba, Brazil

Section 1

Introduction

Chapter 1

Atypical and Anaplastic Meningiomas: Diagnosis and Treatment

Erasmo Barros da Silva Jr, Gustavo Simiano Jung, Joseph Franklin Chenisz da Silva and Ricardo Ramina

Abstract

The aim of this chapter is to describe the usefulness of surgical technologies such as neuronavigation, intraoperative MRI, fluorescence-guided surgery and intraoperative monitoring as a tool do make neurosurgical procedures to brain tumors more safe and effective. The main topics to be explored are: history of the specific technique, indications and contra indications, description of the technique, real case examples, pros and cons. The focus on the discussion besides practical aspects is going to be relevant literature regarding impact of their use in avoidance of complications, improve in survival rates, cost-effectiveness, some tips and tricks acquired in the experience of our department.

Keywords: neurosurgical procedures, brain neoplasms, neuronavigation, fluorescence-guided surgery, magnetic resonance imaging

1. Introduction

Meningiomas originate from specialized meningothelial cells called arachnoid cap cells and correspond about up to 26% of all intracranial lesions. According to the World Health Organization (WHO), meningiomas are grouped in grade I (benign), grade II (atypical), and grade III (anaplastic) [1, 2]. This classification reflects the risk of recurrence and aggressive growth. Although uncommon, atypical corresponds to 4.7 to 20% of all meningiomas, while anaplastic for 1–2.8% [3, 4]. Symptomatology varies according to intracranial location and may be related to seizures and/or intracranial hypertension.

The standard treatment of grade II and grade III meningiomas involve total/radical resection, respecting Simpson score, followed by adjuvant therapy with irradiation and, eventually, chemotherapy [5, 6]. Despite the treatment efforts, the evolution of aggressive meningiomas remains unsatisfactory due to the high rates of local recurrence and/or tumor progression [7]. These patients frequently underwent multiple surgical approaches during the course of the disease, increasing the rates of postoperative complications as infection or CSF leakage.

With the continuous improvement of molecular and immunochemistry analysis, the paradigm for treatment of these tumors has been changing. In this chapter, the current management of aggressive/malignant meningiomas focusing on the new discovers in genetic/molecular and radiotherapy field is discussed.

2. Materials and methods

In our database, we reviewed all meningiomas operated between 2012 and 2017 in our institution to describe the epidemiologic characteristics of atypical and anaplastic subtypes, as well as an illustrative case focusing on the treatment and long-term follow-up. Also, literature was reviewed based on the WHO (2016) classification guided through genetic/molecular findings.

3. Results

A total of 170 new diagnosed patients with intracranial meningiomas underwent microsurgical resection at the Neurological Institute of Curitiba (INC) between January 2012 and June 2017. A total of 94 (55%) tumors were classified as skull base tumors, 58 (34%) convexity, 10 (5.8%) parasagittal, and 8 (4.7%) falcine lesions.

In our series, 76.4% (130) of patients were female. Only six (3.5%) patients had atypical/anaplastic tumors with mean age of 53 years (**Table 1**). Simpson grade I resection (total tumor removal including resection of the underlying bone and associated dura mater) was achieved in all patients with malignant histology, and radiotherapy was reserved for progression. Only one patient with atypical meningioma received upfront radiotherapy because of high Ki-67 index. Any case of skull base meningioma exhibited progression to malignant subtypes in this series.

	Patient 1	Patient 2	Patient 3	Patient 4	Patient 5	Patient 6
Gender	F	M	M	F	F	F
Age	57	58	36	62	65	44
Topography	Parasagittal	Parasagittal	Convexity	Convexity	Convexity	Parasagittal
Histology at 1st resection (WHO)	Grade I	Grade I	Grade I	Grade I	Grade I	Grade I
1st resection (Simpson)	Grade I	Grade I	Grade I	Grade I	Grade I	Grade I
Time to evolution	7m (anaplastic)	26m (anaplastic)	9m (anaplastic)	-	-	16 yrs (atypical)
Radiotherapy modality after anaplastic diagnosis	EBRT	EBRT	EBRT	-	EBRT	EBRT

Table 1.
Malignant meningioma at INC (2012–2017).

4. Illustrative case

58-year-old male has sporadic new onset headache, and magnetic resonance imaging (MRI) evidences enhanced parasagittal homogenous mass tumor with surrounding edema (**Figure 1**). Simpson grade I resection (**Figure 2**) was achieved at surgery, and histopathology confirmed atypical meningioma.

Immunohistochemistry of the first sample proved the trend toward malignant progression, with Ki-67 index of 70% in hot spots. Only focal positiveness for progesterone receptor was seen. Because of high Ki-67 index, adjuvant external beam radiotherapy (EBRT) was added to the treatment.

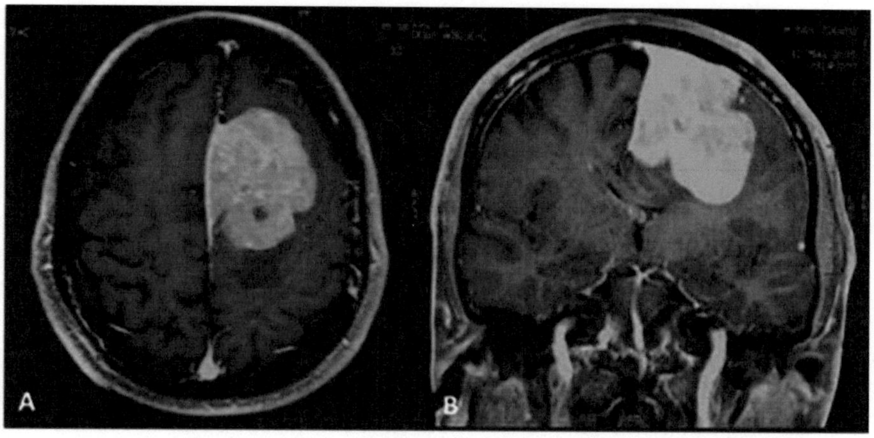

Figure 1.
(A) Post-gadolinium-DTPA axial and coronal. (B) T1-weighted gradient echo (FSPGR) sequence with large parasagittal meningioma with partial occlusion of superior sagittal sinus.

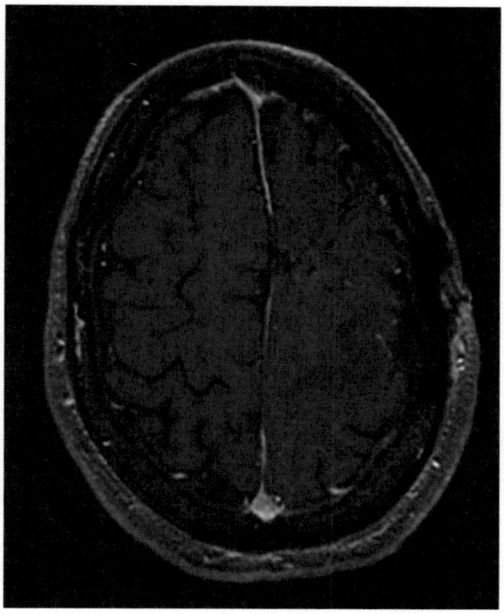

Figure 2.
Postoperative MRI with post-gadolinium-DTPA axial T1-weighted gradient echo (FSPGR) sequence exhibiting complete resection of parasagittal meningioma.

After 1 year follow-up, recurrence at posterior border of previous surgical field was seen, and another gross total resection was necessary (**Figure 3**). The tumor expressed the same imaging characteristics of first analysis, with homogeneous contrast enhancement and peritumoral edema. Histopathological analyses confirmed again an atypical histology. At this time, chemotherapy with octreotide was introduced without response.

After 2 years from the first surgery, another recurrence was seen. At MRI, changes in previous pattern were seen with heterogeneous contrast enhancement and central necrosis (**Figure 4**). After another Simpson grade I tumor removal, progression to anaplastic meningioma was confirmed.

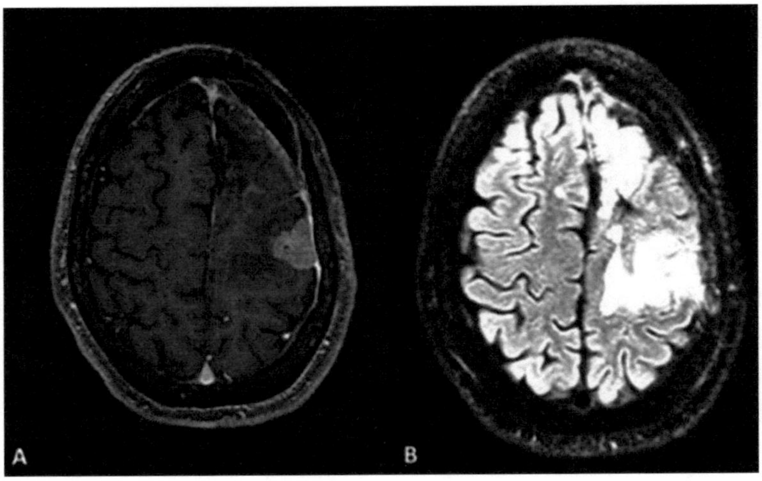

Figure 3.
One-year-follow-up. (A) MRI. Axial post-gadolinium-DTPA T1-weighted gradient echo (FSPGR). (B) Flair sequences evidencing tumor recurrence adjacent to previous resection with the same features of original tumor.

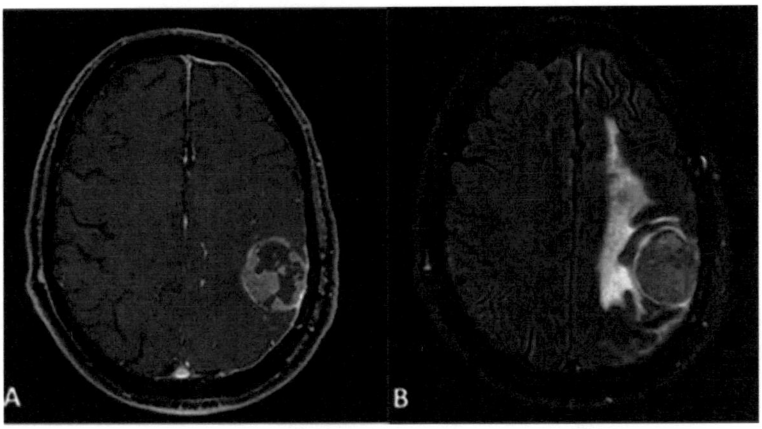

Figure 4.
Axial post-gadolinium-DTPA. (A) T1-weighted gradient echo (FSPGR) showing irregular contrast enhancement and tumoral necrosis. (B) Axial FLAIR magnetic resonance evidencing extensive peritumoral edema with changes in radiological aspect from original tumor.

In comparative analyses, immunohistochemistry evidenced an increase in Ki-67 index from 70 to 90% of the cells. The epithelial membrane antigen (EMA), focal positive at first analysis, now expressed diffuse negativeness. Reduction in progesterone receptor expression was also documented.

Later, there was tumor progression again in two more occasions in an interval of 8 months. Progressive neurological impairment and seizures due to motor cortex/eloquent area involvement/gliosis were seemed, and tumor resection with extensive dural removal was performed both times (**Figures 5** and **6**). The patient underwent salvage irradiation, as the last recurrence was far from the original lesion. Two months after adjuvant treatment, the patient evolved with neurological worsening, dying due to clinical complications.

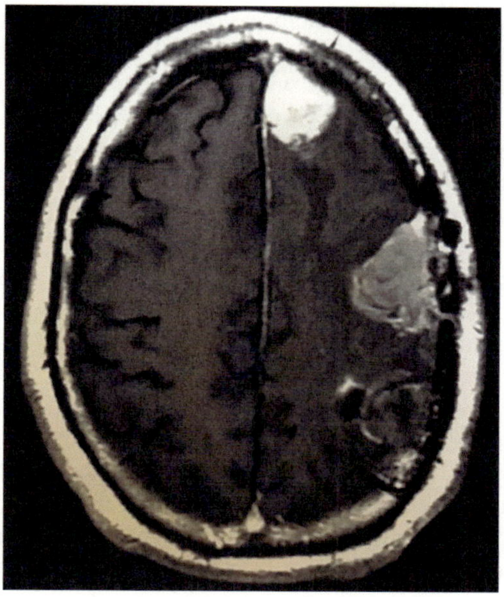

Figure 5.
Axial post-gadolinium-DTPA. (A) T1-weighted gradient echo (FSPGR) showing tumor progression in multiple sites.

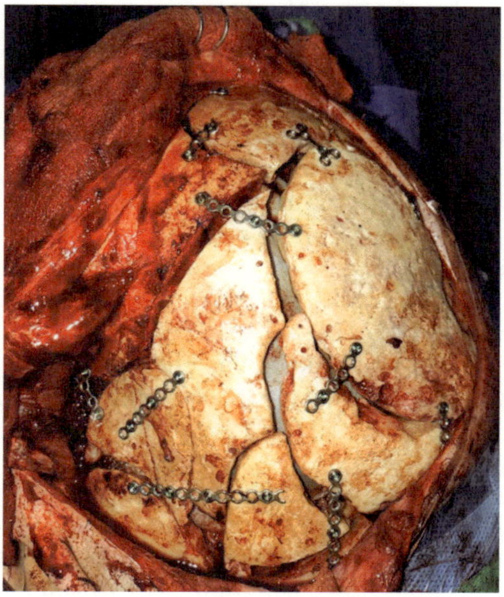

Figure 6.
Intraoperative image showing the skull after multiple craniotomies.

5. Discussion

About 90% of meningiomas are benign grade I tumors. Atypical meningiomas are uncommon (4.7–20% of all meningiomas), while anaplastic meningiomas account for only 1–2.8% of all meningiomas [1–4].

The WHO (2016) classification included brain invasion to the previous histological characteristic (4–19 mitotic figures and 3 of 5 histologic features): increased cellularity, small cells (tumor clusters with high nuclear/cytoplasmic ratio), prominent nucleoli, and sheeting (loss of whorling or fascicular architecture and spontaneous necrosis) in the diagnosis of atypical meningiomas.

Anaplastic meningiomas are diagnosed with 20 or more mitotic figures and presence of frank sarcomatous or carcinomatous histology [3].

Despite of diagnostics criteria, the exact mechanism through how benign meningiomas progress to malignant subtypes remains unclear. Several molecular and genetic hypotheses have been postulated, but the real significance of these alterations is still speculative [8].

Evidence-based literature suggests that the extent of surgical resection, accordingly to Simpson grade system, is the most important prognostic factor for good outcome among those patients harboring malignant meningioma [9].

In our series those cases, with atypical or anaplastic subtypes at primary surgery, demonstrated better response to Simpson grade I resection and adjuvant radiotherapy than those cases that progressed from grade I subtype. Some genetic alteration related to progression, as previously reported in literature, can probably explain different evolution among tumors expressing the same histology like in these series [8, 10, 11].

Among those with atypical and anaplastic histology, tumor size and female gender have been related to poor outcome and presence of radiological features such as heterogeneous enhancement, peritumoral edema, and cyst formation, and absence of calcification have been implicated with lower median recurrence-free survival [9, 12].

In the illustrative case, the tumor progression was followed by changes in radiological characteristics and immunohistochemical pattern. Possibly, in this case, the first immunohistochemistry analysis evidenced some characteristics of aggressiveness. In this scenario, Czonka et al. have previously published the utility of p53 gene expression and Ki-67 index in predicting meningioma progression [13].

Maximal safe resection with dural margins and bone hyperostosis removal stills the main point in the treatment of meningiomas, possibly reducing rates of progression and/or improving progression-free survival [14].

Radiotherapy is a special topic in the treatment of malignant meningiomas. Increase from 15 to 80% in 5 year progression-free survival was reported when EBRT was added to surgical resection for anaplastic meningioma. No consensus exists for atypical meningiomas, and EBRT has mostly been reserved for recurrence and progression [15, 16].

Due to the possibility of margin inclusion in irradiation field with EBRT, radiosurgery is no longer indicated for malignant meningiomas. However, Lubgan et al. have reported excellent results with stereotactic radiotherapy when used as an adjuvant after gross total resection or as definitive treatment regime [17].

In the illustrative case, the lower progesterone receptor expression and higher Ki-67 index could probably predict the chance of progression and help in earlier adjuvant decision.

Several chemotherapy agents have been used for atypical and anaplastic meningiomas refractory to surgery and radiotherapy. In the largest revision, Kaley et al. found 47 publications using different chemotherapy agents (hydroxyurea, temozolomide, irinotecan, interferon-alpha, mifepristone, octreotide analogues, megestrol acetate, bevacizumab, imatinib, erlotinib, and gefitinib) with an average 6 month progression-free survival of 26%, concluding that the available chemotherapy agents provide poor outcomes for refractory malignant meningiomas [18].

6. Conclusion

Atypical and anaplastic meningiomas remain challenging diseases, and no effective treatment is current available. Against literature evidence, we presume that the biological signature of this specific tumor is more important for evolution than previously reported prognostic factor. In this scenario, new studies aiming objective analyses of immunohistochemistry patterns and genetic profile of meningiomas are probably the next step for the comprehension of such complex neurosurgical pathology.

Author details

Erasmo Barros da Silva Jr[1]*, Gustavo Simiano Jung[2], Joseph Franklin Chenisz da Silva[3] and Ricardo Ramina[4]

1 Department of Neurosurgery/Division of Neurooncology, Instituto de Neurologia de Curitiba, Curitiba, Paraná, Brazil

2 Department of Neurosurgery/Division of Skull Base, Instituto de Neurologia de Curitiba, Curitiba, Paraná, Brazil

3 Neurosurgery Resident, Instituto de Neurologia de Curitiba, Curitiba, Paraná, Brazil

4 Head of Department of Neurosurgery, Instituto de Neurologia de Curitiba, Curitiba, Paraná, Brazil

*Address all correspondence to: erasmo-inc@uol.com.br

IntechOpen

© 2018 The Author(s). Licensee IntechOpen. This chapter is distributed under the terms of the Creative Commons Attribution License (http://creativecommons.org/licenses/by/3.0), which permits unrestricted use, distribution, and reproduction in any medium, provided the original work is properly cited.

References

[1] Modha A, Guttin PH. Diagnosis and treatment of atypical and anaplastic meningiomas: A review. Neurosurgery. 2005;**57**(3):538-550

[2] Yang SY, Park CK, Park SH, Kim DG, Chung YS, Jung HW. Atypical and anaplastic meningiomas: Prognostic implications of clinicopathological features. Journal of Neurology, Neurosurgery, and Psychiatry. 2008;**79**(5):574-580. DOI: 10.1136/jnnp.2007.121582

[3] Komori T, Sasaki H, Yoshida K. Revised WHO classification of tumor of the central nervous system: Summary of the revision and perspective. No Shinkei Geka. 2016;**44**(8):625-635. DOI: 10.11477/mf.1436203347

[4] Komotar RJ, Iorgulescu JB, Raper DM, Holland EC, Beal K, Bilsky MH, et al. The role of radiotherapy following gross-total resection of atypical meningiomas. Journal of Neurosurgery. 2012;**117**(4):679-686. DOI: 10.3171/2012.7.JNS112113

[5] Hasan S, Young M, Albert T, Shah AH, Okoye C, Bregy A, et al. The role of adjuvant radiotherapy after gross total resection of atypical meningiomas. World Neurosurgery. 2015;**83**(5):808-815. DOI: 10.1016/j.wneu.2014.12.037

[6] Sun SQ, Hawasli AH, Huang J, Chicoine MR, Kim AH. An evidence based treatment algorithm for the management of WHO grade II and III meningiomas. Neurosurgical Focus. 2015;**38**(3):E3. DOI: 10.3171/2015.1.FOCUS14757

[7] Walcott BP, NAhed BV, Brastianos PK, Loeffler JS. Radiation treatment for WHO grade II and III meningiomas. Frontiers in Oncology. 2013;**3**:227

[8] Pérez-Magán E, Campos-Martín Y, Mur P, Fiaño C, Ribalta T, García JF, et al. Genetic alteration associated with progression and recurrence in meningiomas. Journal of Neuropathology and Experimental Neurology. 2012;**71**(10):882-893. DOI: 10.1097/NEN.0b013e31826bf704

[9] Nanda A, Bir SC, Konar S, Maiti T, Kalakoti P, Jacobsohn JA, et al. Outcome of resection of WHO grade II meningioma and correlation of pathological and radiological predictive factors of recurrence. Journal of Clinical Neuroscience. 2016;**31**:112-121. DOI: 10.1016/j.jocn.2016.02.021

[10] Bujko M, Machnicki MM, Grecka E, Rusetska N, Matyja E, Kober P, et al. Mutational analysis of recurrent meningioma progressing from atypical to Rhabdoid subtype. World Neurosurgery. 2017;**97**:754.e1-754.e6. DOI: 10.1016/j.wneu.2016.10.047

[11] Yuzawa S, Nishihara H, Tanaka S. Genetic landscape of Meningiomas. Brain Tumor Pathology. 2016;**33**(4):237-247

[12] Jääskeläinen J, Haltia M, Servo A. Atypical and anaplastic meningiomas: Radiology, surgery, radiotherapy, and outcome. Surgical Neurology. 1986;**25**(3):233-242

[13] Csonka T, Murnyák B, Szepesi R, Bencze J, Bognár L, Klekner A, et al. Assessment of candidate immunohistochemical prognostic markers of meningioma recurrence. Folia Neuropathologica. 2016;**54**(2):114-126

[14] Aizer A, Bi W, Kandola M, Lee E, Nayak L, Rinne M, et al. Extent of resection and overall survival for patients with atypical and malignant meningioma. Cancer. 2015;**121**(24):4376-4381

[15] Dziuk TW, Woo S, Butler EB, Thornby J, Grossman R, Dennis WS, et al. Malignant meningioma: An

indication for initial aggressive surgery and adjuvant radiotherapy. Journal of Neuro-Oncology. 1998;**37**(2):177-188

[16] Jung GS, Ramina R, da Silva EB Jr, Neto MC. Diagnosis and predictors of treatment outcomes in Meningiomas with atypical or anaplastic histology. Jornal Brasileiro de Neurocirurgia. 2016;**27**(2):100-104

[17] Lubgan D, Rutzner S, Lambrecht U, Rössler K, Buchfelder M, Eyüpoglu I, et al. Stereotactic radiotherapy as primary definitive or postoperative treatment of intracranial meningioma of who grade II and III leads to better disease control than stereotactic radiotherapy of recurrent meningioma. Journal of Neuro-Oncology. 2017;**134**:407-416. DOI: 10.1007/s11060-017-2540-7

[18] Kaley T, Barani I, Chamberlain M, McDermott M, Panageas K, Raizer J, et al. Historical benchmarks for medical therapy trials in surgery and radiation refractory meningioma: A RANO review. Neuro-Oncology. 2014;**16**(6):829-840. DOI: 10.1093/neuonc/not330

Section 2

Diagnosis and Treatment Modalities

Chapter 2

Molecular Diagnostics and Pathology of Major Brain Tumors

Frank Y. Shan, E. Castro, Amelia Sybenga, Sanjib Mukherjee, Erxi Wu, Karming Fung, The Li, Ekokobe Fonkem, Jason H. Huang and A. Rao

Abstract

Tumors of central nervous system (CNS) account for a small portion of tumors of human body, which include tumors occurring in the parenchyma of brain and spinal cord as well as their coverings. The following chapter covers some new development in some major brain tumors in both pediatric and adult populations, as well as some uncommon but diagnostic and management challenging tumors.

Keywords: gliomas, astrocytomas, oligodendrogliomas, mixed oligoastrocytomas, WHO (World Health Organization), WHO grades, medulloblastomas (MBs), midline diffuse astrocytoma, diffuse intrinsic pontine gliomas (DIPG), hemangioblastomas (HMBs), metastatic renal cell carcinoma (RCC), formalin-fixed, paraffin-embedded (FFPE), H3 K27M mutation, immunohistochemical (IHC) stain, fluorescence in situ hybridization (FISH)

1. Introduction

Tumors of central nervous system (CNS) include the tumors of the brain and spinal cord, as well as their covers. Those tumors are uncommon tumors, accounting for approximately 1% of all human body tumors. They can be divided into primary or secondary/metastatic tumors, benign or malignant tumors, based on the WHO classification; brain tumors are assigned into four grades, from Grade 1 very benign tumor to Grade IV highly malignant tumors (see below). By location, those tumors can be divided into extra-axial tumors (outside brain/spinal cord parenchyma), such as meningiomas, and intra-axial tumors (inside brain/spinal cord parenchyma), such as gliomas. Diagnosis of brain tumors is primarily based on the WHO Classification of Tumors of CNS; this expert consensus scheme was first completed in 1979 and then revised in 1993, 2000, and 2016. This scheme is currently the most widely utilized by neuropathologists worldwide for typing and grading the CNS tumors [1]. Neoplasms, especially those malignant ones, are biologically characterized by noncontrolled tumor cell proliferation; this uncontrolled growth is best explained by recently discovered EGFR (epidermal growth factor receptor) mutations, which mutations result in uncontrolled signal transduction downward to nuclei without ligand binding to the receptor and led to unlimited cell proliferation.

 IntechOpen

During the last two decades, a lot of gene mutations are identified, especially in the oncology field, which has been helpful for the development of new generation of antitumor medication focusing on the mutated gene products. As a matter of fact, those target treatments have already archived tremendous successes in the oncology field. For example, gefitinib, erlotinib, and afatinib are the current targeted medications against EGFR-mutated non-small-cell lung cancers, which already show great clinical success.

The following chapter is going to review some development in brain tumors, especially the recent understanding of adult gliomas and pediatric medulloblastomas, as well as some other uncommon tumors for their molecular diagnosis and genetic subgrouping.

2. Molecular diagnosis of adult gliomas

Glial tumors comprise approximately 25–30% of primary CNS tumors [1] and represent a spectrum ranging from low-grade, benign to the highly aggressive, malignant tumors. They are broadly classified by glial cell type of origin and determined by histology with or without the use of immunohistochemistry (IHC), which is then used to provide a WHO grade (see **Table 1**) [1]; however, histology has not been able to accurately predict response to treatment or clinical outcomes, and it is not uncommon for many of these tumors with nearly identical histologic features to have very different outcomes. As a result of these observations, and like many malignancies (lung and colorectal carcinoma for example), there has been increasing interest in attempting to further classify these tumors based on their molecular expression. With that interest there is an increase in available published data regarding these molecular alterations and a subsequent increase in the availability of myriad testing modalities; some of which are now considered well established, while others are not. In an era of test utilization awareness and rising healthcare costs, this phenomenon frequently leads to confusion regarding which tests should be utilized, how those tests should be interpreted, and how they should be reported, in order to best guide treatment and predict outcomes in this patient population [2].

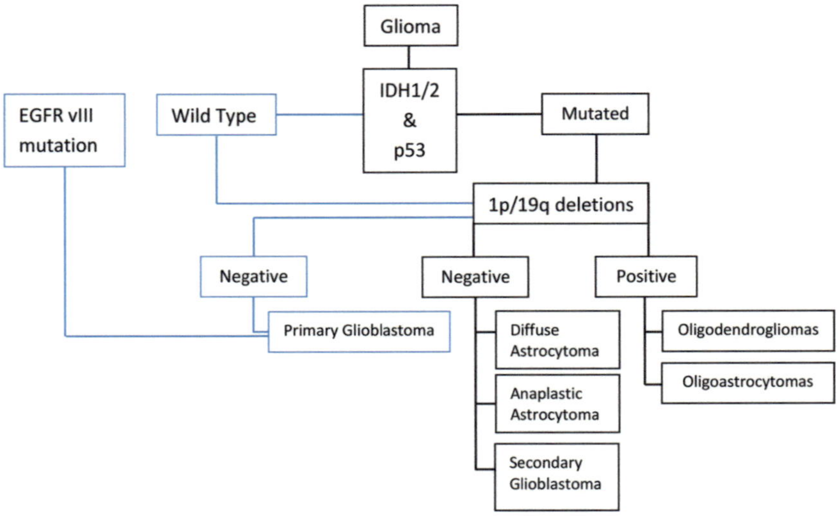

Table 1.
Molecular genetic map for the development of adult gliomas.

We will discuss here the well-established molecular concepts, touch briefly on the evolving molecular discoveries, and provide a testing algorithm (see **Table 1**).

Glioblastoma (GBM) is the most aggressive primary CNS malignancy, WHO Grade IV [1]. Despite decades of research and multiple new treatment modalities, little progress has been made in terms of substantial improvements of patients' outcomes, with the average long-term survival being measured in months rather than years [3]. However, this research has illuminated a complex series of molecular pathways and events that is improving our understanding of the pathophysiology of this aggressive entity.

2.1 LOH 10q

Loss of heterozygosity (LOH) at chromosome 10q occurs with high frequency in both primary and secondary GBMs, occurring in both in approximately 60–80% of cases [4]. Although this is an interesting primary event in the development of GBM of either type, because of its high frequency, it is not useful in distinguishing one from the other. Instead, GBM is currently subclassified by its molecular alterations into primary and secondary GBM, based on the presence or absence of IDH1/IDH2 and/or TP53 mutations [4]. EGFR status is also being increasingly used in this context.

2.2 IDH1/IDH2

Isocitrate dehydrogenase-1 (IDH1) is an NADP-dependent enzyme found in the cytoplasm responsible for the conversion of isocitrate to α-ketoglutarate and thereby producing NADPH, which reduces reactive oxygen species. IDH2 is similarly present in mitochondria. Their exact role in tumorigenesis is poorly understood; however, it is thought that mutations in this enzyme result in increased oxidative stress and subsequent carcinogenesis. It is therefore not surprising that this mutation is not found in primary GBMs, rather secondary GBMs that have progressed from a less aggressive tumor, and diffuse and anaplastic astrocytomas (WHO Grade II and III, respectively). IDH mutations are found with high frequency in the majority of astrocytomas, oligodendrogliomas, mixed gliomas, and secondary GBMs but not in pilocytic astrocytomas or primary GBMs. The most common mutation in IDH1 is a point mutation (arginine to histidine at codon 132), termed IDH1-R132H. IDH2 mutations (IDH2 172) represent only 3–5% of IDH mutations and are more commonly found in oligodendrogliomas. IDH mutations have also shown an association with hypoxia-inducible factor 1 alpha (HIF1), associated with upregulation of vascular endothelial growth factor (VEGF). Recent study indicates that low-grade astrocytomas with wild-type IDH1 behavior as glioblastoma clinically, suggesting again the importance of IDH1 mutation status in gliomas. IDH1 mutation can be detected by IHC, and commercially available mouse antihuman monoclonal antibody by Dianova with clone name H09 is a favored antibody to IDH1 R132H by most neuropathologists.

Secondary glioblastomas confer a significantly better prognosis than those arising de novo (primary GBM), and occur in a younger age group with a history of pervious low grade gliomas [4]. Because primary and secondary GBMs cannot be distinguished morphologically, IDH1/2 mutation testing can be utilized for this task, allowing for better prognostication. IDH1/2 is commercially available as a reverse transcriptase PCR (RT-PCR) test. Although an IHC stain is available, it is not as sensitive to the less common variants of IDH1/2 mutation; however, it can be highly useful in the detection of single tumor cells in diffuse gliomas [5–7]. It is important to note that the role of IDH1/2 mutations in predicting response to therapy is still debated. It appears that the mutation confers an increased response to radiation therapy, while others show an increased response with chemotherapy as well. Response appears to be multifactorial, dependent not only on the type of therapy, but also on the time of that therapy in relation to surgical resection [8]. Importantly, IDH mutations serve as a surrogate marker for secondary GBMs [9]. This testing should be performed in conjunction with TP53 and Ki67 on all GBMs, and considered standard of care.

2.3 P53

P53 is a cyclin-dependent kinase responsible for tumor suppression through prevention of cell replication. Mutations in p53 in malignant tumors are well established in the literature, with greater than 50% of cancers showing p53 loss of function mutations [10]. P53 is more commonly a missense mutation that results in accumulation of the protein in the cytoplasm, resulting in diffuse, strong nuclear staining by IHC; however, alternate mutations in p53 can show complete absence of staining or cytoplasmic staining only, whereas the wild type (unmutated) p53 will show weak to moderate, patchy positivity [11].

Most tumors that express p53 mutations typically have a more aggressive course than those that do not; however, this relationship has not been established in GBMs. Currently, no statistically significant difference has been established that GBMs with p53 mutations have a worse prognosis than those that do not [12]. The utility of p53 in GBMs, similar to IDH1/2 mutation status, is as additional evidence of a secondary GBM, rather than a primary GBM, as p53 mutations are far less frequent in primary GBMs, and, when present, likely represent secondary or late events associated with increasing genetic instability [4].

2.4 Epidermal growth factor receptor (EGFR)

EGFR is a member of the transmembrane tyrosine kinase receptor family that activates MAPK and PIK3 pathways resulting in cell proliferation. EGFR testing started to gain particular popularity due in part to the development of tyrosine kinase inhibitors (TKIs) and after a 2010 study by Verhaak et al. that attempted to further subclassify GBMs based on multiple molecular markers [15]. EGFR amplification confers more aggressive behavior and poorer outcomes, autophosphorylating the PIK3 pathway, leading to increased growth, angiogenesis, metastatic potential, and reduced apoptosis [16]. In contrast to secondary GBMs, epidermal growth factor receptor (EGFR) overexpression has been demonstrated in 36% of primary GBMs, with 70% of those showing amplification. It exists most commonly as the mutation EGFR variant 3 (EGFRvIII), which has deletion of exons 2 and 7 [17]. EFGRvIII mutation testing is performed with RT-PCR [17]. Unlike other malignancies where tyrosine kinase inhibitor (TKI) immunotherapy has shown wide successes, GBMs frequently do not respond, showed only a partial response, or develop rapid resistance to TKIs. This most often attributed to PTEN loss earlier in the EGFR pathway [4]. EGFR amplification or mutation in this context can be utilized, when present, as further support of a primary GBM over a secondary GBM.

In addition to the discovery of multiple molecular alterations in MET, PDGFRA, NF1, PTEN, PIK3 and CDKN2A/B, and several others, studies have discovered alterations of several microRNAs, which are also a field of current study. Importantly, none of these have been well established in terms of either their prognostic significance or their impact on treatment response, and several studies have shown contradictory results. This likely can be attributed to the marked heterogeneity of glial tumors, particularly GBMs. It is not currently recommended to add these markers to a broader profile until their clinical significance can be better established.

2.5 1p/19q co-deletion

Chromosome arms 1p and 19q deletions are the most characterized genetic aberrations of oligodendrogliomas, with up to 80% of classical oligodendrogliomas (WHO Grade II) and 60% of anaplastic oligodendrogliomas (WHO Grade III) [18, 19]. Although it seems unclear what impact these deletions have on cellular function, there are two identified roles for testing these deletions: the first is as a diagnostic marker for oligodendroglial tumors and the other as an indicator of response to treatment. One study demonstrated that the presence of complete or partial co-deletion of 1p and 19q conferred a significantly increased response to chemotherapy, and prolonged disease-free survival time, compared with those tumors with deletion of only one or the other chromosomal arm, regardless of histologic subtype [20], consistent with other studies, including mixed tumors. Due to the significant clinical implications for the presence of this gene, 1p/19q co-deletion testing should be performed on all glial tumors with or without oligodendroglial features since a small percentage (5%) of morphological astrocytomas are with 1p/19q co-deletion, which may confer a slightly better prognosis for the patients. Testing is available by both FISH and for LOH by real-time PCR. Evaluation of both chromosomal arms in their entirety is recommended due to molecular variability.

2.6 MGMT methylation

O^6-methylguanine-DNA methyltransferase (MGMT) codes for MGMT repair protein, and methylation of this gene, which results in suppression and decreased expression of the MGMT protein, confers a significant survival benefit in patient treated with combined radiation and temozolomide therapy. MGMT methylation occurs in all types of gliomas and with frequency in primary and secondary GBMs and oligodendrogliomas (60–93%). In predicting a positive response to treatment, MGMT methylation also predicts an increased survival benefit. In lower-grade gliomas, MGMT methylation confers an increased response to radiation monotherapy, which is not well understood [9].

Methylation-specific PCR is the testing modality of choice and is widely available. An alternative is pyrosequencing, which shows high sensitivity, but is now less frequently used. Other testing modalities, such as western blot and IHC, have fallen into disuse due to issues with false-positive results.

Table 1 summarizes the current understanding of tumorigenesis for adult gliomas.

3. Molecular diagnosis of diffuse midline gliomas with H3 K27M mutation

It has been recognized for almost 20 years among pediatric neuro-oncologists that neuroimaging study defined diffuse intrinsic pontine gliomas (DIPG) had a very poor prognosis independent of histological grade (if biopsied). In that case, biopsy is most of the time considered unnecessary until recent identification of potential drug targets for individualized therapy has led to reevaluation of this approach [22]. Recent genomic analysis has demonstrated that specific genetic alterations drive distinct subsets of glial neoplasm of the central nervous system, dependent not only on tumor-type but also on the site of origin and patient age. Like this diffuse midline gliomas, with somatic mutations of the H3F3A and HIST1H3B gene encoding the histone H3 variants, H3.3 and H3.1, were recently identified in high-grade gliomas arising in the thalamus, pons, and spinal cord of children and young adults; those tumors are named as diffuse midline gliomas with H3 K27M mutation [23].

Brainstem tumors affect primarily children and young adults. Each year, around 300–400 cases of brainstem tumors are diagnosed in the United States, and diffuse intrinsic pontine glioma (DIPG) accounts approximately 80% of these tumors [24]. DIPG has been recently categorized by WHO classification as high-grade (Grade IV) diffuse midline gliomas with H3 K27M mutation. It carries a poor prognosis, and only 1% of the patients live 5 years after diagnosis.

Clinically, diffuse midline gliomas result in brainstem dysfunction and the obstruction of cerebrospinal fluid (CSF) flow. The patients suffer from difficulty in ocular movements, weakness of facial muscles, sudden hearing problem, swallowing difficulty, muscle spasticity, clonus, and bladder dysfunction, along with multiple cranial neuropathies and ataxia.

Diagnosis of diffuse midline gliomas is initiated through imaging primarily by MRI scans indicating hypointense (T1) or hyperintense (T2) lesions, enhancing or non-enhancing after administration of contract agents. Biopsy is a standard procedure for establishing the molecular and histopathological diagnoses. This tumor shows many histopathological features of glioblastoma such as pseudopalisading necrosis and microvascular proliferation, in addition to H3 K27M positive by immunohistochemical (IHC) stain (**Figure 1**).

Unlike many other adult gliomas, debunking surgery, with gross total resection (GTR) of the tumor, is not a treatment of choice for diffuse midline gliomas, mainly due to the location of the tumors. The brainstem regulates critical bodily functions, and therefore surgical resection without damaging the vital area of the brainstem is almost impossible. Surgery is indicated only for biopsy of the tumor and to relieve the hydrocephalus that may happen in a small fraction of cases. Currently, patients are treated primarily with radiation and adjuvant chemotherapy with temozolomide.

In diffuse midline gliomas with H3 K27 mutation, lysine in 27th position of tail of Histone 3.3 is replaced by methionine. Histones are the alkaline protein that provides a scaffold, around which DNA wraps. Solomon and colleague have observed that H3K37M mutation in pontine gliomas occurred at a much younger age (median 7 years of age) than gliomas of the thalamus (median age, 24 years) or spinal cord (median age, 25 years) [23]. The H3 K27M-positive gliomas have also been reported in adult in the brainstem [25]. High-grade gliomas with H3 K27M mutation may have additional mutations (WHO, 2016). These mutations are observed to occur in the critical genes, regulating cell divisions including cell cycle checkpoints and chromatin remodeling. The most frequent additional mutation noted is tumor suppressor p53, which is noted in an estimated half of the H3 K27M

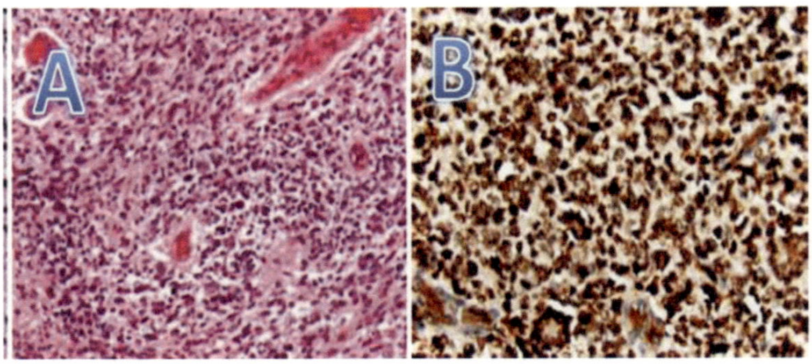

Figure 1.
(A) Grade IV midline glioblastoma and (B) IHC + for H3 K27M mutation.

midline gliomas. Amplification of platelet-derived growth factor alpha (PDGFRA), critical for cell survival and proliferation, is observed in about 30% of the H3 K27M tumors. Cyclin-dependent kinases 4 and 6 are reported to be amplified in 20% of the tumors, and homozygous deletion of cyclin-dependent kinase inhibitor 2A/2B is noted in 5% of the H3 K27M gliomas. Mutation of activin A receptor type-1 (AVCR1) is noted in 20% of H3 K27M gliomas. A mutation of protein phosphatase 1D (PPM1D) and amplification of MYC/PVT1 may present separately, in 15% of the H3 K27M gliomas [1]. In addition, histone H3 K27M mutation is found mutually exclusive with IDH1 mutation and EGFR amplification, rarely co-occurred with BRAF-V600E mutation, and was commonly associated with p53 overexpression, ATRX loss (except in pontine gliomas), and monosomy 10 [23].

These mutations could provide us with a better understanding of the disease process and could potentially lead to the development of a better treatment strategy for this deadly disease. As a matter of fact, at least two clinical trials are underway with small molecule inhibitor of the histone demethylase, which showed some promising result [23].

4. Molecular subgroups of medulloblastomas

Medulloblastoma is the most common malignant brain tumor of cerebellum in childhood, although it rarely happens in adult patients, too. It is an embryonal neuro-epithelial tumor arising in the cerebellum or dorsal brainstem, which is a major cause of morbidity and mortality in pediatric brain tumor patients [27, 28], and was designed as WHO Grade IV neoplasm [1]. Histologically, medulloblastoma is a prototypical embryonal tumor, consisting of densely packed small round undifferentiated blue tumor cells with mild to moderate nuclear pleomorphism and a high mitotic count, mostly with Homer-Wright rosettes, and shows different morphological variants, such as desmoplastic/nodular, large cell, and anaplastic, etc., with predominantly neuronal differentiation and tendency to metastasize via CSF pathways [1] (**Figures 2** and **3**).

4.1 Morphologic features of medulloblastomas

Several morphological variants of MBs are recognized, alongside the classic tumor: desmoplastic/nodular MB, MB with extensive nodularity, and large-cell/anaplastic MB. A dominant population of undifferentiated cells with a high nuclear-to-cytoplasmic ratio and active mitotic figures is a common feature [1] (**Figures 2** and **3**). Classic MB composed of sheets of undifferentiated small blue

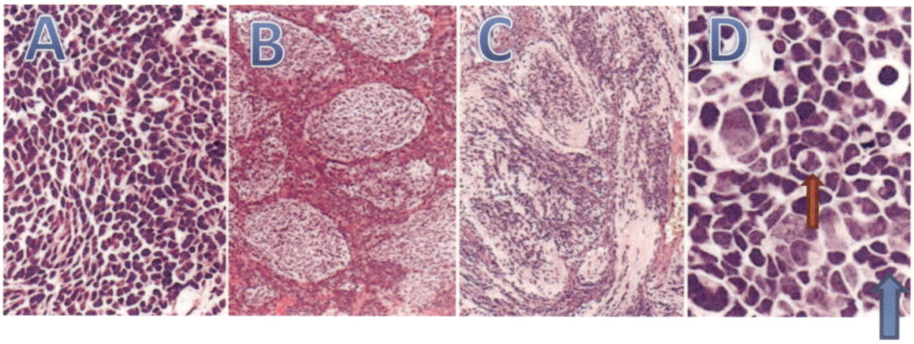

Figure 2.
Histopathology of MBs. (A) Classic type, 70%; (B) nodular, 10%; (C) extensive nodularity, 3%; and (D) large cell/anaplastic, 15% (arrow nuclear molding, blue; wrapping, red).

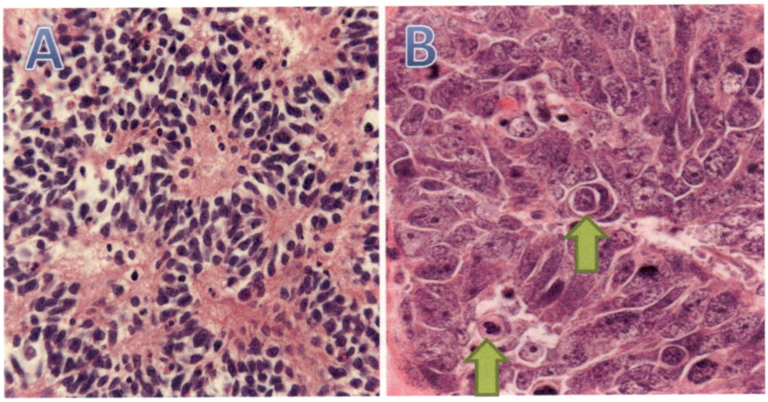

Figure 3.
Histopathology of MBs. (A) Homer Wright rosettes and (B) nuclear wrapping (hugging), arrow, in large-cell/anaplastic MBs.

tumor cells with Homer-Wright rosette formations and/or palisading tumor cells forming a pseudoglandular feature, easily found mitoses and apoptosis. Other histological variants include desmoplastic MB, which contains abundant reticulin and collagen, characterized with nodular reticulin-free zones (pale islands). The nodules have reduced cellularity, a rarified fibrillar matrix and marked nuclear uniformity. A rare histologic type of MB is the so-called large-cell MB, which is composed completely or partially of cells with large, round nuclei and prominent nucleoli, commonly with large areas of necrosis. The large-cell MB sometimes resembles the rhabdoid/atypical teratoid (RT/AT) tumors of cerebellum, but its cytoplasm lacks globular hyaline inclusions and is diffusely reactive for synaptophysin, neurofilament protein, and vimentin and negative for epithelial membrane antigen, cytokeratins, and smooth-muscle actin by immunohistochemical (IHC) stains [1]. Most often associated with large-cell MB is anaplastic MB, which is characterized by angular, crowded, pleomorphic nuclei in large cells, sometimes with nuclear molding and wrapping (**Figure 3**), mitosis, and apoptosis, as well as prominent nucleoli. It has been noted for a long time that morphology of MBs was related to patient's prognosis and that those MBs with extensive nodularity are with better prognosis, while the large-cell/anaplastic MBs are usually associated with worse clinical outcomes (**Figure 1**).

Additional study indicates that poor survival outcome was significantly associated with chromosome 17p loss (loss of tumor suppressor) and high expression of oncogenes c-myc (MYCC) or N-myc (MYCN) [1].

Due to the highly heterogeneous nature of the MB, and complication caused by aggressive treatments, a more specific subgrouping of this tumor is becoming more and more important for clinical judgment.

Molecular studies from multiple groups around the world found that medulloblastoma is not a single disease but comprises a collection of clinically and molecularly diverse subgroups. Current consensus made in a 2010 meeting at Boston agrees that there are four principal subgroups of medulloblastomas [27, 28] termed as WNT, SHH, Group 3, and Group 4.

Two of these subgroups, characterized by either activated WNT or SHH signaling pathway, are thought to play prominent roles in the pathogenesis. Two other non-WNT/non-SHH groups are more closely related to each other and even produced additional different numbers of subgroups within these groups of MBs, pending additional evidence to further classify them [27, 28].

4.1.1 MB, WNT subgroup

The best known subgroup of the medulloblastoma is the WNT subgroup due to its very good long-term prognosis, compared to other subgroups. WNT indicates the wingless signaling pathway.

WNT medulloblastomas are characterized by upregulation of the canonical WNT signaling pathway, which results in translocation of β-catenin to the nucleus. About two-thirds harbor a CTNNB1 mutation. Mutations in other pathways, such as APC and AXIN1, have been reported in the absence of a CTNNB1 mutation but are much less frequent [27]. The extent of β-catenin nuclear immunoreactivity in these WNT pathway MBs always amounts to more than a third of the total tumor area and is clearly different from the situation where very few scattered β-catenin nucleopositive cells, representing less than 2% of tumor cells, are evident. Assays for CTNNB1 mutation and monosomy 6, which occurs in nearly all WNT pathway MBs, have helped to establish the status of tumors in these immunohistochemical categories [27]. There is a close association between a WNT pathway immunophenotype and CTNNB1 mutation or monosomy 6, predicting a good outcome for medulloblastomas with these genetic abnormalities [27].

More than 90% of WNT subgroup medulloblastoma patients achieved long-term survival, with those patients whose death is due to more complications of therapy or secondary tumors rather than due to recurrent WNT medulloblastomas. Germline mutations of the WNT pathway inhibit APC predispose to Turcot syndrome, which includes a proclivity to medulloblastoma; in addition, somatic mutations of CTNNB1 encoding β-catinin have been found in sporadic medulloblastomas [27]. These strong germline and somatic genetic data support an etiological role for canonical WNT signaling in the pathogenesis of this group of tumors and lead to the nomenclature of "WNT subgroup of medulloblastomas."

Almost all WNT medulloblastomas have classic histology, which often described as having CTNNB1 mutations, with nuclear labeling for β-catenin by immunohistochemical stain, and monosomy 6 (deletion of one copy of chromosome 6 in tumor cells). Medulloblastomas with large-cell/anaplastic features have also been reported in the WNT subgroup, although they appear to maintain the excellent prognosis associated with the WNT subgroup. Which of monosomy 6, nuclear staining for β-catenin, mutation of CTNNB1, immunohistochemical staining for DKK1, or a transcriptional signature that clusters with other WNT tumors should be used as a gold standard for the diagnosis of WNT medulloblastomas awaits further validation on large cohorts of well-characterized medulloblastomas.

WNT-activated MBs account for approximately 10% of all MBs, most of them present in children aged between 7 and 14 years, but they can also occur in young adults. Genetically, besides CTNNB1, genes that are recurrently mutated in WNT-activated MBs include TP53, SMARCA4, and DDX3X [1].

4.1.2 MB, SHH subgroup with TP53 mutant

The SHH group of MBs are named after the sonic hedgehog signaling pathway. In large series of tumors, SHH-activated MBs tend to have similar transcriptome, methylome, and microRNA profiles. SHH pathway activation in TP53-mutant tumors is associated with amplification of GLI2, MYCN, or SHH. Mutations in PTCH1, SUFU, and SMO are genetically absent. Large-cell/anaplastic morphology and chromosome 17p loss are also common in SHH-activated and TP53-mutant tumors. Patterns of chromosome shattering known as chromothripsis are often present.

SHH-activated tumors account for approximately 30% of all MBs and originate from rhombic lip-derived cerebellar granule neuron precursors. SHH-activated and TP53-mutant MBs are rare and generally found in children aged 4–17 years. Clinical outcomes in patients with SHH-activated and TP53-mutant tumors are very poor [1].

4.1.3 MB, SHH subgroup, with TP53 wild type

SHH pathway activation in TP53 wild-type tumors can be associated with germline or somatic mutation in the negative regulations PTCH1 or SUFU, as well as activating somatic mutations in SMO or (rarely) amplification of GLI2. Desmoplastic/nodular MBs and MBs with extensive nodularity are always included in the SHH-activated group, but tumors with a SHH signaling pathway can also have a classic or large-cell/anaplastic morphology, particularly in older children. Patients with SHH-activated and TP53 wild-type MBs are generally children aged <4 years, adolescents, or young adults. In addition to genetic changes activating SHH signaling, mutations in DDX3X or KMT2D and amplification of MYCN or MYCL are sometimes seen, as are deletions of chromosomal arms 9q, 10q, and 14q. Clinical outcomes in patients with SHH-activated tumors are variable [1].

4.2 Epidemiology

Research data from 1973 to 2007 suggested MB incidence rates of 0.6 cases per 1 million children aged 1–9 years and 0.6 cases per 1 million adults aged >19 years. SHH-activated MBs in general show a bimodal age distribution, being most common in infants and young adults, with a male-female ratio of approximately 1.5:1. In contrast, SHH-activated and TP53-mutant tumors are generally found in children aged 4–17 years. In one study including 133 SHH-activated MBs, 28 patients (21%) had a TP53 mutation, and the median age of these patients was approximately 15 years [1].

4.2.1 Groups 3 and 4/non-WNT and non-SHH groups

Groups 3 and 4 MBs are usually called "the non-WNT/non-SHH groups." They share some of the similarities in both clinical presentation and molecular profiling. Most tumors in these groups display classical histology. The large-cell/anaplastic and desmoplastic histologies are present but at a lower frequency. The age of onset is distributed in both groups with most patients are children; they are relatively uncommon in infants and adults. Although both groups have similar frequency of metastasis, Group 3 shows poor prognosis, while Group 4 shows intermediate prognosis. Non-WNT and non-SHH tumors account for approximately 60% of all MBs and typically have classic histopathological features [1].

One characteristic similarity between Groups 3 and 4 is both subgroups are enriched for expression of genes involved in photoreceptor differentiation, and they express high level of OTX2 and FOXG1B, well-known oncogenes of MB. However, Group 3 is distinguished by its enriched gene signatures functioning in cell cycle, protein biosynthesis, glutamate receptor signaling, and p38 mitogen-activated protein kinase (MMAPK) pathway, while Group 4 is overrepresented by genes involved in neuronal differentiation, development, cytoskeleton organization, etc.

In addition, isochromosome 17q (I17q) represents the most common structural abnormality in Groups 3 and 4. Other chromosomal alteration identified in these subgroups includes gain of 7 and 18q and loss of 8 and 11q. The major difference between these two groups is the enrichment of MYC amplification in Group 3, which is very rarely observed in Group 4, as well as in WNT and SHH. Another difference is the enrichment of chromosome X loss in Group 4, found in 80% female MBs in Group 4.

The signaling pathway or biological programs driving the tumorigenesis of Groups 3 and 4 still remain largely unknown, although some reports suggest that disruption of chromatin genes associated with histone methylation may be a critical event driving Groups 3 and 4 tumor developments.

4.3 Medulloblastoma molecular subgroups: immunophenotypes and histopathological associations

After multigroup extensive researches, the development and validation of immunohistochemical stains to define molecular subgroups of MBs finally archived, with 4 immunohistochemical staining marker identified in order to MBs subgrouping, which can be used in FFPE tissue and greatly improve the routine pathological diagnosis process for these types of tumors. Four immunostaining markers were selected for pathological subgrouping of MBs: they are β-catenin, GAB1, filamin A, and YAP1 [27].

4.3.1 SHH pathway MBs

Combined immunoreactivities for GAB1, filamin A, and YAP1, indicating a SHH profile, were found in 31% of MBs, including all desmoplastic tumors. Desmoplastic MBs constituted 54% of SHH pathway tumors, and classic and large-cell/anaplastic tumors contributed 29 and 17%, respectively. While non-desmoplastic SHH tumor generally showed widespread and strong immunoreactivities for GAB1, YAP1, and filamin A, all three types of desmoplastic tumors displayed stronger staining for these proteins within internodular regions. Immunoreactivities for filamin A and YAP1 in SHH tumors were always strong and generally widespread. This was not always the situation for GAB1 immunoreactivity; no more than weak cytoplasmic staining for GAB1 was seen in a few non-desmoplastic SHH tumors ($n = 6$). These tumors were all strongly immunopositive for filamin A and YAP1, which acted to confirm the SHH phenotype [27].

4.3.2 WNT pathway MBs

Antibodies to β-catenin for identifying WNT tumors effective on formalin-fixed and paraffin-embedded (FFPE) tissue are well established in the diagnostic laboratory [27]. Widespread intermediate or strong cytoplasmic β-catenin immunoreactivity was a feature of nearly all MBs in the series; very few showed only patchy weak cytoplasmic staining for this antigen. WNT pathway MBs were identified by nuclear, as well as cytoplasmic, immunoreactivity for β-catenin (**Figure 4**). WNT pathway MBs defined by these types of nuclear β-catenin immunoreactivity also express filamin A. Typically, this was patchy staining and less intense than that seen in SHH tumors. Strong and widespread nuclear immunoreactivity for YAP1 was also a feature of WNT pathway tumors. This distinctive combination of β-catenin, filamin A, and YAP1 immunoreactivities robustly confirmed the status of MBs in this molecular subgroup. WNT tumors contributed 14% of all MBs in this study. Nearly all WNT pathway MBs were classic tumors. Large-cell/anaplastic tumor ($n = 2$, 6%) was exceptional among WNT tumors, while desmoplastic MBs were not represented [27].

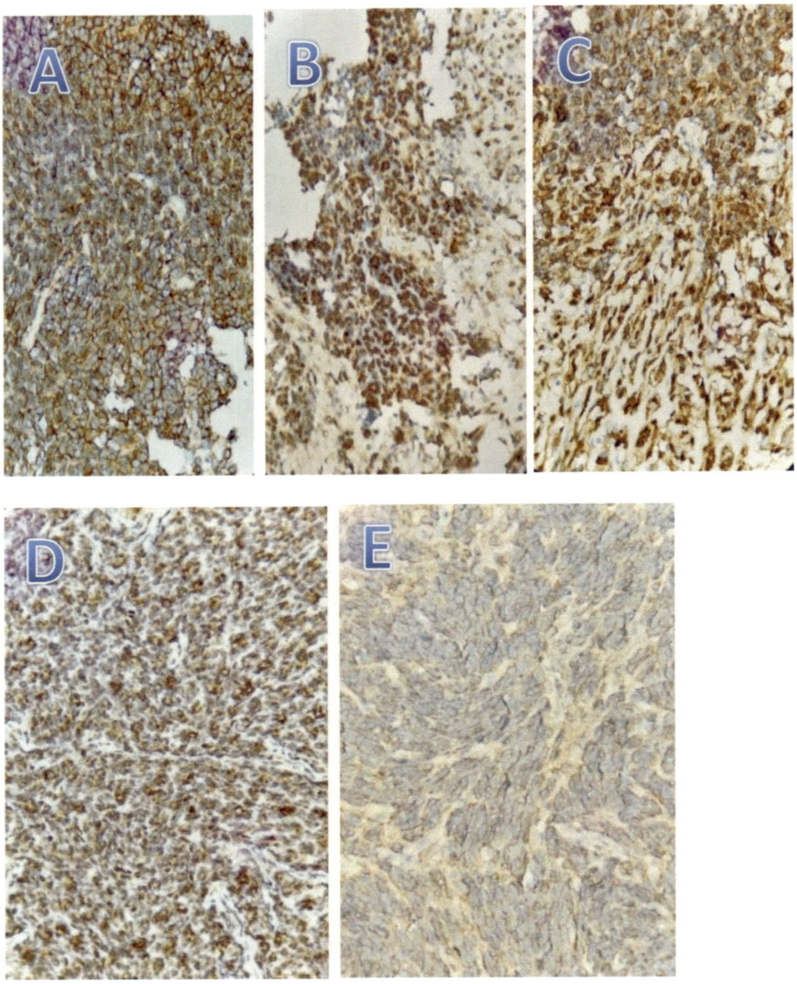

Figure 4.
β-Catenin IHC stain with both nuclear and cytoplasmic positive (A and C), GAB1 stain positive (B), YAP1 (D), and filamin A (E).

4.3.3 Non-SHH/WNT MBs

MBs (N = 130, 55%) falling outside the SHH and WNT categories displayed cytoplasmic, but not nuclear, immunoreactivity for β-catenin. Tumor cells were negative for GAB1 and YAP1. In general, tumors in this category were also immunonegative for filamin A, though very weak and patch immunoreactivity for this antigen was evident in rare non-SHH/WNT MBs (n = 9), which were classified as such on the basis of the panel of immunoreactivities. Intrinsic vascular elements were immunopositive for YAP1 and filamin A, providing an internal control. This subgroup of MBs was dominated by classic tumors (92%), including all non-desmoplastic nodular tumors and all but one MB that contained small clusters of densely packed neurocytic cells, the exception being a WNT tumor. Large-cell/anaplastic tumors made up the remainder (n = 11) [27].

4.3.4 Metastatic MBs

Despite four subgroups, metastatic MBs exist among all subgroups although the incidence of metastatic dissemination is higher in Group 3 and 4 than WNT and

IHC marker	IHC stain for MBs	MBs subgrouping	
	WNT	SHH	Non-WNT/non-SHH
β-Catenin	N+, C+, ¼ focal	C+	C+
GAB1	Neg	C+	Neg
Filamin A	C+	C+	Neg
YAP1	N+, C+	N+, C+	Neg

N+, nuclear staining positive; C+, cytoplasmic staining positive; SHH, Sonic Hedgehog.

Table 2.
Subgrouping MBs by immunohistochemical stains.

SHH [33]. Metastatic MBs occur in approximately 40% of all MBs at diagnosis and are associated with poorer prognosis [34]. In 2001, McDonald et al. [35] identified potential therapeutic targets, e.g., PDGFRα PDGFR for metastatic MBs using expression array analysis. However, Gilbertson and Clifford [36] found that the probe McDonald used for PDGFRα was PDGFRβ. They further demonstrated that PDGFRβ is overexpressed in metastatic MB. Then, Kohane and his co-workers did an interesting experiment and found that genomically, human MBs were closest to mouse P (postnatal) 1-P10 cerebella, and normal human cerebella were closest to mouse P30-P60. Metastatic human MBs were highly associated with mouse P5 cerebella (non-metastatic human MB with mouse P7 cerebella). PDGFRα is highly expressed in P5; PDGFRβ in P7 [37]. However, which isoform of PDGFRs plays a role in metastatic MBs kept controversial. Ten years later, we demonstrated that PDGFRα inhibits while PDGFRβ promotes MB cell proliferation and cell survival as well as cell invasion [38], highlighting that PDGFRβ may serve as a potential therapeutic target for metastatic MBs and warrants further investigation, including clinical studies.

Table 2 summarizes the IHC staining for subgroups of MBs.

5. Hemangioblastoma, metastatic renal cell carcinoma, and von Hippel-Lindau disease

Hemangioblastoma (HMB) is a benign, slow-growing, WHO grade I tumor, most likely occurs in cerebellum, brainstem, and spinal cord. Most hemangioblastomas are cystic on neuroimaging with intramural nodule. Histologically, the tumor has two major components, one is tightly packed capillary small vessels, and another is so-called stromal cells with low-grade nuclei, foamy cytoplasm, and no prominent nucleoli. Mitosis and necrosis are absent. But some degenerative features are often present [1].

On the other hand, cerebellum is a favorite location for metastatic renal cell carcinoma (RCC). Histologically, most RCC has clear cytoplasm with rich vascular supply, but slightly higher-grade nuclei mostly have small nucleoli.

Due to the similarity in histology and the same preference location, 70% of HMBs occur in sporadic forms, while approximately 30% of HMBs are associated with the inherited von Hippel-Lindau disease. The VHL tumor suppressor gene is inactivated both in VHL-associated cases and in most sporadic cases [1].

Von Hippel-Lindau disease (VHL) is a familial disorder predisposing patients to cysts and hypervascular neoplasm of multiple organs, including the CNS, eye, kidneys, adrenal medulla, pancreas, inner ear/temporal bone, and epididymis.

VHL is an autosomal dominant disorder, with roughly 20% of patients presenting as sporadic cases with no family history. The VHL tumor suppressor gene maps to chromosome 3p25 and includes three highly conserved exons [31].

VHL-associated disease includes [31] the following:

- Retinal hemangioblastomas (40–60%)
- CNS hemangioblastomas (60–80%)
- Endolymphatic sac tumor (2–11%)
- Pheochromocytomas (10–25%)
- Pancreatic cysts or islet tumors (60–80%)
- Renal cysts and RCCs (30–60%)
- Papillary cystadenomas of the epididymis (20–60%)

Solitary and especially multiple HMBs are diagnostic hallmarks of VHL. Roughly 75% are infratentorial, mainly involving the cerebellum. The rest of them are found

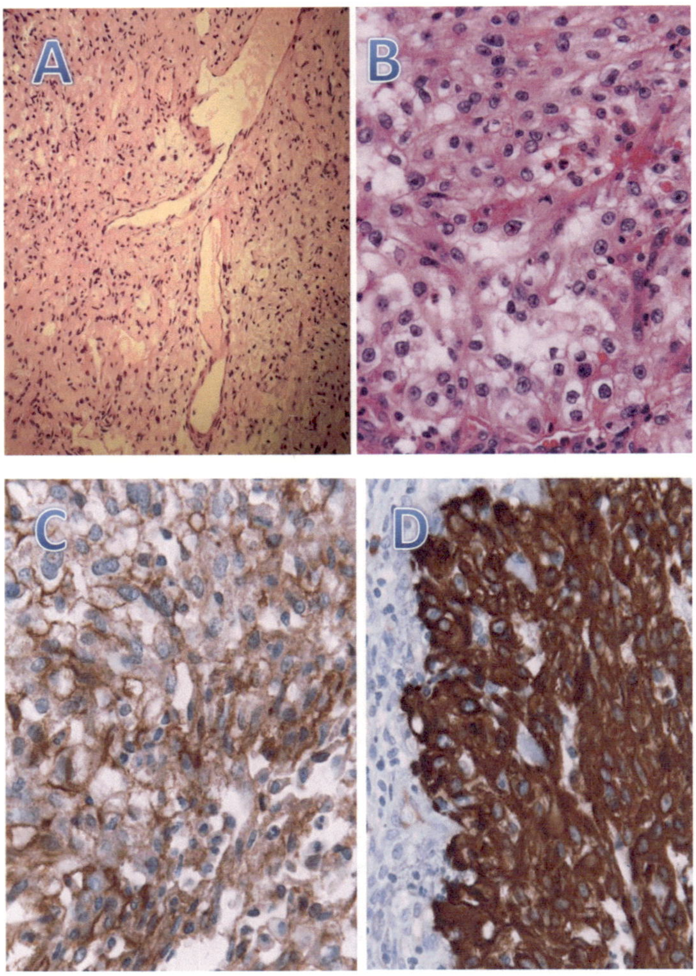

Figure 5.
Hemangioblastoma, H&E stain ×200, with low-grade nuclei and foamy stromal cells (A); metastatic RCC with clear cytoplasm, larger nuclei, and prominent nucleoli H&E stain ×400 (B); and RCC is immunoreactive for CD10 (C) and cytokeratin (D).

in the spinal cord, brainstem, and lumbosacral nerve roots. Supratentorial HMBs are extremely rare. Of interest, only about 25–30% of cerebellar HMBs are seen in VHL patients, whereas this fraction rises to 80% in the spinal cord [1].

It is may be those two tumors share the same chromosome locus of 3p25; they have some histological overlapping as well as the same preference of anatomic location (cerebellum); HMB and metastatic RCC are two tumors almost always request differentiation diagnosis, since one is benign and another is malignant, both carry different prognoses, and this two tumors become "forever differential diagnosis" for most diagnostic neuropathologists. Luckily, a simple small panel of immunohistochemical (IHC) stain would easily resolve this puzzle. HMB is negative for cytokeratin but positive for inhibin and 2D40, while RCC will be positive for cytokeratin, CD10, and PAX-8 and negative for inhibin [31] (**Figure 5**).

6. Summary

Research work in the last two decades discovered lots of genetic alterations in human brain tumors. More work will be done to further facilitate the diagnosis and classification. A recent proposal is suggested by using the epigenomics, like methylation status, to enhance brain tumor classification [32]. A new clinical trial with medication focusing on the IDH1 mutation is underway now; as more and more research data collected, we believe more effective treatment options will be developed in the near future. For a more detailed review on the molecular neuropathology of brain tumors, please refer to Ref. [39].

Author details

Frank Y. Shan[1,2*], E. Castro[1], Amelia Sybenga[1], Sanjib Mukherjee[3], Erxi Wu[2], Karming Fung[4], The Li[5], Ekokobe Fonkem[2], Jason H. Huang[2] and A. Rao[1]

1 Department of Anatomic Pathology, Scott & White Medical Center, College of Medicine, Texas A&M University, Temple, TX, USA

2 Department of Neurosurgery, Scott & White Medical Center, College of Medicine, Texas A&M University, Temple, TX, USA

3 Vasicek Cancer Center, Scott & White Medical Center, College of Medicine, Texas A&M University, Temple, TX, USA

4 Department of Pathology, Oklahoma University Medical Center, Oklahoma City, OK, USA

5 Department of Pathology, Guangdong General Hospital, Guangzhou, Guangdong, China

*Address all correspondence to: yshan918@gmail.com

IntechOpen

© 2018 The Author(s). Licensee IntechOpen. This chapter is distributed under the terms of the Creative Commons Attribution License (http://creativecommons.org/licenses/by/3.0), which permits unrestricted use, distribution, and reproduction in any medium, provided the original work is properly cited.

References

[1] Louis DN, Ohgaki H, Wiestler OD, Cavenee WK. WHO Classification of Tumours of the Central Nervous System. Revised 4th ed. Lyon: International Agency for Research on Cancer; 2016

[2] Ballester LY, Huse JT, Tang G, et al. Molecular classification of adult diffuse gliomas: Conflicting IDH1/IDH2, ATRX, and 1p/19q results. Human Pathology. 2017;**69**:15-22. DOI: 10.1016/j.humpath.2017.05.005

[3] Lieberman F. Glioblastoma update: Molecular biology, diagnosis, treatment, response assessment, and translational clinical trials. F1000 Research. 2017;**6**:1892. DOI: 10.12688/f1000research.11493.1

[4] Ohgaki H, Kleihues P. Genetic pathways to primary and secondary glioblastoma. The American Journal of Pathology. 2007;**170**:1445-1453. DOI: 10.2353/ajpath.2007.070011

[5] Capper D, Zentgraf H, Balss J, et al. Monoclonal antibody specific for IDH1 R132H mutation. Acta Neuropathologica. 2009;**118**:599-601. DOI: 10.1007/s00401-009-0595-z

[6] Capper D, Weissert S, Balss J, et al. Characterization of R132H mutation-specific IDH1 antibody binding in brain tumors. Brain Pathology (Zurich, Switzerland). 2010;**20**:245-254. DOI: 10.1111/j.1750-3639.2009.00352.x

[7] Kato Y, Jin G, Kuan C-T, et al. A monoclonal antibody IMab-1 specifically recognizes IDH1R132H, the most common glioma-derived mutation. Biochemical and Biophysical Research Communications. 2009;**390**:547-551. DOI: 10.1016/j.bbrc.2009.10.001

[8] Cohen AL, Holmen SL, Colman H. IDH1 and IDH2 mutations in gliomas. Current Neurology and Neuroscience Reports. 2013;**13**:345. DOI: 10.1007/s11910-013-0345-4

[9] van den Bent MJ, Dubbink HJ, Marie Y, et al. IDH1 and IDH2 mutations are prognostic but not predictive for outcome in anaplastic oligodendroglial tumors: A report of the European Organization for Research and Treatment of Cancer Brain Tumor Group. Clinical Cancer Research: An Official Journal of the American Association for Cancer Research. 2010;**16**:1597-1604. DOI: 10.1158/1078-0432.CCR-09-2902

[10] Ozaki T, Nakagawara A. Role of p53 in cell death and human cancers. Cancers. 2011;**3**:994-1013. DOI: 10.3390/cancers3010994

[11] Yemelyanova A, Vang R, Kshirsagar M, et al. Immunohistochemical staining patterns of p53 can serve as a surrogate marker for TP53 mutations in ovarian carcinoma: An immunohistochemical and nucleotide sequencing analysis. Modern Pathology: An Official Journal of the United States and Canadian Academy of Pathology, Inc. 2011;**24**:1248-1253. DOI: 10.1038/modpathol.2011.85

[12] England B, Huang T, Karsy M. Current understanding of the role and targeting of tumor suppressor p53 in glioblastoma multiforme. Tumour Biology: The Journal of theInternational Society for Oncodevelopmental Biology and Medicine. 2013;**34**:2063-2074. DOI: 10.1007/s13277-013-0871-3

[13] Gielen GH, Gessi M, Hammes J, et al. H3F3A K27M mutation in pediatric CNS tumors: A marker for diffuse high-grade astrocytomas. American Journal of Clinical Pathology. 2013;**139**:345-349. DOI: 10.1309/AJCPABOHBC33FVMO

[14] Venneti S, Santi M, Felicella MM, et al. A sensitive and specific

histopathologic prognostic marker for H3F3A K27M mutant pediatric glioblastomas. Acta Neuropathologica. 2014;**128**:743-753. DOI: 10.1007/s00401-014-1338-3

[15] Verhaak RGW, Hoadley KA, Purdom E, et al. Integrated genomic analysis identifies clinically relevant subtypes of glioblastoma characterized by abnormalities in PDGFRA, IDH1, EGFR, and NF1. Cancer Cell. 2010;**17**:98-110. DOI: 10.1016/j.ccr.2009.12.020

[16] Taylor TE, Furnari FB, Cavenee WK. Targeting EGFR for treatment of glioblastoma: Molecular basis to overcome resistance. Current Cancer Drug Targets. 2012;**12**:197-209

[17] Mansouri A, Karamchandani J, Das S. Molecular genetics of secondary glioblastoma. In: De Vleeschouwer S, editor. Glioblastoma. Brisbane (AU): Codon Publications; 2017. Available from: http://www.ncbi.nlm.nih.gov/books/NBK469981/ [Accessed: June 1, 2018]

[18] Jeuken JWM, von Deimling A, Wesseling P. Molecular pathogenesis of oligodendroglial tumors. Journal of Neuro-Oncology. 2004;**70**:161-181. DOI: 10.1007/s11060-004-2748-1

[19] Chaturbedi A, Yu L, Linskey ME, et al. Detection of 1p19q deletion by real-time comparative quantitative PCR. Biomarker Insights. 2012;**7**:9-17. DOI: 10.4137/BMI.S9003

[20] McNamara MG, Jiang H, Lim-Fat MJ, et al. Treatment outcomes in 1p19q co-deleted/partially deleted gliomas. Canadian Journal of Neurological Sciences. 2017;**44**:288-294. DOI: 10.1017/cjn.2016.420

[21] Scheie D, Cvancarova M, Mørk S, et al. Can morphology predict 1p/19q loss in oligodendroglial tumours? Histopathology. 2008;**53**:578-587. DOI: 10.1111/j.1365-2559.2008.03160.x

[22] Von Burern AO, Karremann M, Gielen GH, Benesch M, Fouladi M, van Vuurden DG, et al. A suggestion to introduce the diagnosis of "diffuse midline glioma of the pons, H3 K27 wildtype (WHO grade IV)". Acta Neuropathologica. 2018

[23] Solomon DA, Wood MD, Tihan T, Bollen AW, Gupta N, Phillips JJJ, et al. Diffuse midline gliomas with histone H3-K27M mutation: A series of 47 cases assessing the spectrum of morphologic variation and associated genetic alterations. Brain Pathology. 2016;**26**(5):569-580

[24] Warren KE. Diffuse intrinsic pontine glioma: Poised for progress. Frontiers in Oncology. 2012;**2**:205

[25] Daoud EV, Rajaram V, Cai C, Oberle RJ, Martin GR, Raisanen JM, et al. Adult brainstem gliomas with H3K27 M mutation: Radiology, pathology, and prognosis. Journal of Neuropathology and Experimental Neurology. 2018;**77**(4):302-311. DOI: 10.1093/jnen/nly006

[26] Hofman LM, Veldhuijzen van Zanten SEM, Colditz N, Baugh J, Chaney B, Hofmann M, et al. Clinical, radiologic, pathologic, and molecular characteristics of long-term survivors of diffuse intrinsic pontine glioma (DIPG): A collaborative report from the international and European society for pediatric oncology DIPG registries. Journal of Clinical Oncology. 2018

[27] Ellison DW, Dalton J, Kocak M, Nicholson SL, Fraga C, Neale G, et al. Medulloblastoma: Clinicopathological correlations of SHH, WNT, and non-SHH/WNT molecular subgroups. Acta Neuropathologica. 2011;**121**(3):381-396

[28] Taylor MD, Northcott PA, Korshunov A, Remke M, Cho YJ, Clifford SC, et al. Molecular subgroups of medulloblastoma: The current consensus. Acta Neuropathologica. 2012;**123**:465-472

[29] Ellison DW, Onilude OE, Lindsey JC, Lusher ME, Weston CL, Taylor RE, et al. β-Catenin status predicts a favorable outcome in childhood medulloblastoma. Journal of Clinical Oncology. 2005;**23**:7951-7957

[30] Thompson MC, Fuller C, Hogg TL, Dalton J, Finklestein D, Lau CC, et al. Genomic identifies medulloblastoma subgroups that are enriched for specific genetic alterations. Journal of Clinical Oncology. 2006;**24**:1924-1931

[31] Perry A, Brat DJ. Practical Surgical Neuropathology. Philadelphia, PA, USA: Churchill Livingston/Elsevier; 2010. ISBN: 978-0-443-06982-6

[32] Capper D, Jones DTW, Still M, et al. DNA methylation-based classification of central nervous system tumors. Nature. 2018, 2018;**555**:469-474. DOI: 10.1038/nature26000

[33] Zapotocky M, Mata-Mbemba D, Sumerauer D, Liby P, Lassaletta A, Zamecnik J, et al. Differential patterns of metastatic dissemination across medulloblastoma subgroups. Journal of Neurosurgery. Pediatrics. 2018;**21**(2):145-152. DOI: 10.3171/2017.8.PEDS17264. Epub: December 8, 2017

[34] Miranda Kuzan-Fischer C, Juraschka K, Taylor MD. Medulloblastoma in the Molecular Era. Journal of Korean Neurosurgical Association. 2018;**61**(3):292-301. DOI: 10.3340/jkns.2018.0028. Epub: May 1, 2018

[35] MacDonald TJ, Brown KM, LaFleur B, Peterson K, Lawlor C, Chen Y, et al. Expression profiling of medulloblastoma: PDGFRA and the RAS/MAPK pathway as therapeutic targets for metastatic disease. Nat Genet. 2001;**29**(2):143-52. Erratum. Nature Genetics. 2003;**35**(3):287

[36] Gilbertson RJ, Clifford SC. PDGFRB is overexpressed in metastatic medulloblastoma. Nature Genetics. 2003;**35**(3):197-198

[37] Kho AT, Zhao Q, Cai Z, Butte AJ, Kim JY, Pomeroy SL, et al. Conserved mechanisms across development and tumorigenesis revealed by a mouse development perspective of human cancers. Genes & Development. 2004;**18**(6):629-640

[38] Wang F, Remke M, Bhat K, Wong ET, Zhou S, Ramaswamy V, et al. A microRNA-1280/JAG2 network comprises a novel biological target in high-risk medulloblastoma. Oncotarget. 2015;**6**(5):2709-2724

[39] Velazquez VJE, Brat DJ. Incorporating advances in molecular pathology into brain tumor diagnostics. Advances in Anatomic Pathology. 2018;**25**(3):143-171

Chapter 3

Potential Use of Long Noncoding RNAs as Biomarkers for Astrocytoma

Ruth Ruiz Esparza-Garrido, Alicia Siordia-Reyes, Gerardo Sánchez, Griselda Ramírez and Miguel Velázquez-Flores

Abstract

Noncoding RNAs represent a high proportion of the human genome and regulate gene expression by means of innumerable and unimaginable modes of action. Particularly, long noncoding RNAs have emerged as central regulators of gene expression and alterations on their function have been associated with many types of cancer, such as astrocytomas. Astrocytomas are the most common type of gliomas in the central nervous system, and glioblastoma multiforme is their most aggressive form. Although adult and pediatric astrocytomas exhibit certain molecular similarities, they are considered as distinct molecular entities. Since to date there is no effective treatments for these tumors, different efforts are being made to find molecular tools useful for this purpose. Studies have shown that both tumor and circulating expression of lncRNAs were altered in astrocytoma, which was useful to distinguish the patients with this neoplasia from those without cancer, as well as to determine different prognostic factors related to the disease. According to these studies, different "molecular signatures" of specific lncRNAs were established, and they have a potential use in the medical practice. From a system biological perspective, complex interaction networks, conformed by lncRNAs, microRNAs, mRNAs, and proteins, were elucidated and predicted to control many oncogenic processes.

Keywords: astrocytoma, biomarker, interacting network, lncRNA, microRNA

1. Introduction

Noncoding RNAs (ncRNAs) represent a significant fraction of the human genome [1], and the great diversity and forms of action of these RNA species has put them at the center of biomedical research of diseases, such as cancer [2–4]. LncRNAs are not the exception, and many of them have been proposed as possible diagnostic and prognostic biomarkers for Ast [5]. LncRNAs are RNAs of more than >200 nucleotides in length, which have to meet certain additional criteria to be classified within this category [6]. The evolutionary conservation of lncRNAs among species is poor [7], and they are transcribed by a variety of transcriptional mechanisms [6]. Many cellular processes are regulated by lncRNAs and this could be at both cytoplasmic and nuclear levels, as well as distance by moving them to their target tissues through different bodily fluids, such as blood [8]. LncRNAs exert their functions by establishing interactions with other lncRNA and RNA species, as well as with proteins [9], and changes on their functioning have been associated with cancer and particularly with astrocytomas (Ast) [5].

Gliomas represent 81% of the Central Nervous System (CNS) tumors of which the most common subtypes in adults are glioblastoma multiforme (GBM), anaplastic Ast (AAst), and oligodendrogliomas [10, 11]. In the pediatric counterpart, pilocytic Ast (PAst) is the most common type in pediatric age [11]. According to the new classification of the World Health Organization (WHO), Ast are now classified according to the presence or absence of *IDH1*/*IDH2* mutations, as well as by phenotypic traits and integral diagnoses [12]. Those tumors with *IDH1*/*IDH2* mutations were classified as "diffuse gliomas," a new group that includes diffuse Ast (DAst; Grade II), AAst (Grade III), GBM, and diffuse oligodendrogliomas (Grade I and II) [12]. Meanwhile, pilocytic Ast (PAst; Grade I), subependymal giant cells Ast (Grade I), and pleomorphic xanthoastrocytoma (Grade II) were excluded from the diffuse group, given that they do not have these mutations [12]. Although there are certain molecular similarities between adult and pediatric Ast (p-Ast) [13], their molecular differences are well established and based on this, they are classified as different tumor subtypes [14–17]. Although there have been advances in the Ast study—mainly on adult GBM—, to date, there are very few molecular tools useful for Ast diagnosis, prognosis, and treatment. Essentially, most studies have identified changes on the expression of lncRNAs in both tumor tissues and GBM cell lines, and according to this, some "molecular signatures" have been postulated for the diagnosis and prognosis of Ast. For instance, circulating lncRNAs have allowed the distinction of patients sensitive or resistant to treatments, specifically to temozolomide (TMZ) or radiotherapy [18, 19]. In addition, the establishment of bioinformatic algorithms identified interactome networks in which lncRNAs physically interact with other lncRNAs, as well as with messenger RNAs (mRNAs) and microRNAs (miRNAs), and proteins. These studies have shown that expression changes of lncRNAs could lead to the amplification of the aberrant signals, which in turn could lead to alterations of many signaling pathways and cellular processes [5, 20, 21]. In p-Ast, high expression levels of LINC-ROR (long intergenic nonprotein coding RNA, regulator of reprogramming) were useful to distinguish p-Ast from the control, as well as to identify the GBM from the rest of the Ast grades; this strongly suggests the involvement of LINC-ROR in p-Ast diagnosis and prognosis [5].

2. Astrocytoma

Although the new WHO classification of tumors of the CNS takes into account phenotypic traits, it also takes into account other criteria, such as the genotype and integral diagnoses of the disease [12]. According to this classification, Ast are now classified mainly by the presence or absence of *IDH1*/*IDH2* mutations and based on this, diffuse Ast (DAst; Grade II) and anaplastic Ast (AAst; Grade III), as well as the GBM, and diffuse oligodendrogliomas (Grade I and II) were classified as "diffuse gliomas" [12]. PAst, subependymal giant cells Ast, and pleomorphic xanthoastrocytoma (Grade II) were classified in a different group, because of the absence of *IDH1*/*IDH2* mutations.

2.1 Astrocytomas that lack IDH1 and IDH2 mutations

These tumors have a well circumscribed growth pattern, lack IDH alterations, and they frequently have *BRAF* (pilocytic Ast (Past) and pleomorphic xanthoastrocytoma) and *TSC1*/*TSC2* mutations (subependymal giant cells Ast) (**Table 1**).

PAst are the most common type of Ast in pediatric age and are characterized by their biphasic pattern: compact bipolar cells with Rosenthal fibers, microquistes, and granular bodies (**Figure 1A**). As a general rule, PAst are well-defined tumors

WHO Classification	
Astrocytomas that lack IDH1 and IDH2 mutations	
Pilocytic astrocytoma Subependymal giant cell astrocytoma	WHO grade I
Pleomorphic xanthoastrocytoma	WHO grade II
Diffuse gliomas	
Diffuse astrocytoma, IDH-mutant Gemistocytic astrocytoma, IDH-mutant Diffuse astrocytoma, IDH-wildtype Diffuse astrocytoma, NOS	WHO grade II
Anaplastic astrocytoma, IDH-mutant Anaplastic astrocytoma, IDH-wild type Anaplastic astrocytoma, NOS Anaplastic pleomorphic xanthoastrocytoma	WHO grade III
Glioblastoma GBM, IDH-mutant GBM, IDH-mutant GBM, NOS	
GBM Variants Epithelioid glioblastoma GBM with primitive neuronal component Small cell GBM/Ast Granular cell GBM/Ast	

Table 1.
Astrocytoma classification according to the World Health Organization (2016).

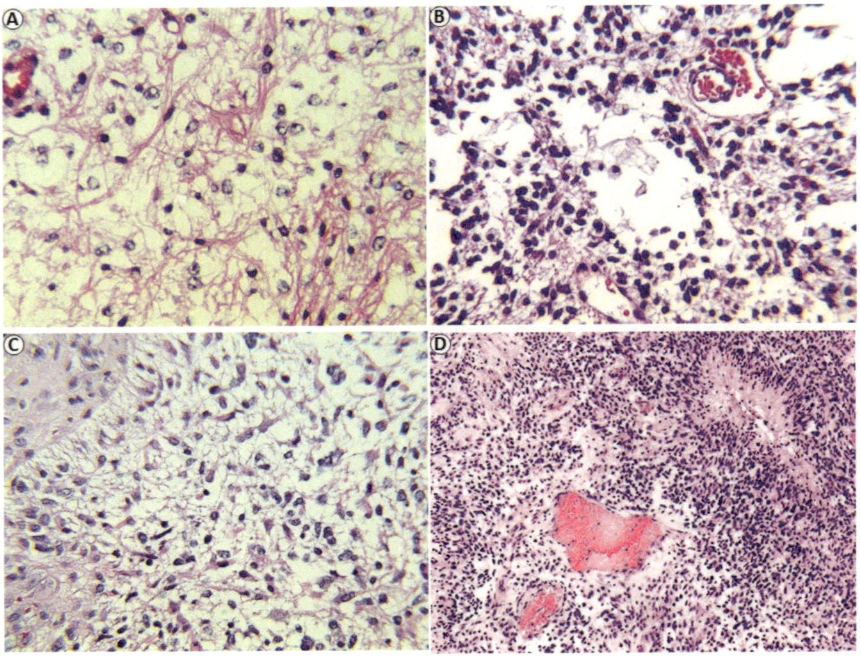

Figure 1.
(A) Pilocytic Ast. Photomicrograph that shows a glioma with astrocytes, which have an elongated cytoplasm and a pilocytic appearance, on a loose stroma (H&E, 40×). (B) Diffuse astrocytoma. Diffuse glioma with cysts and solid areas; the cells are homogenous and do not exhibit atypia (H&E, 40×). (C) Anaplastic astrocytoma. Neoplasia with hypercellularity and nuclear pleomorphism and hyperchromatism. In the upper left, a blood vessel with a glomerular pattern can be seen (H&E, 40×). (D) GBM. Hypercellular glial tumor with diffuse pleomorphism and necrosis; it is delimitated by palisaded cells, which are characteristic of GBM (H&E, 10×). Photomicrographs taken at the pediatric Pathology Service of the Children's Hospital, National Medical Center Century XXI, IMSS.

(**Figure 2A**); so they can be surgically resected without causing damage to the adjacent tissue and they do not progress to more aggressive stages; therefore, PAst are considered as neoplasms of good prognosis.

PAst are developed along the neuroaxis, and they are preferably located in the cerebellum [22–24]. It is important to mention that there are genetic diseases such as neurofibromatosis 1 (*NF-1*), which influences the formation of PAst; approximately 15% of individuals with *NF-1* develop these type of tumors, specifically at the level of the optic nerve [25, 26].

2.2 Diffuse gliomas (tumors with IDH1 and IDH2 mutations)

In the previous WHO classification, diffuse Ast (DAst) were classified as an independent group, but now they are classified along with anaplastic Ast (Aast; Grade III) and glioblastoma (GBM; Grade IV) (**Figures 1B–D** and **2B–D**), as well as with diffuse oligodendrogliomas (Grade I and II) [12]. Although factors such as growth and tumor behavior are still taken into account, the feature that distinguishes them as diffuse gliomas are the *IDH1* and *IDH2* mutations; however, these tumors can be subclassified into the *IDH*-mutant, *IDH*-wildtype, and NOS categories [12].

IDH-wildtype neoplasms constitute a subgroup of uncommon tumors, which are negative for mutant R132H *IDH1* protein and genic mutations for *IDH1* (codon 132) and *IDH2* (codon 172). Importantly, DAst (WHO Grade II) and AAst (WHO Grade III) can be confused with gangliogliomas and *IDH*-wildtype GBM [27, 28].

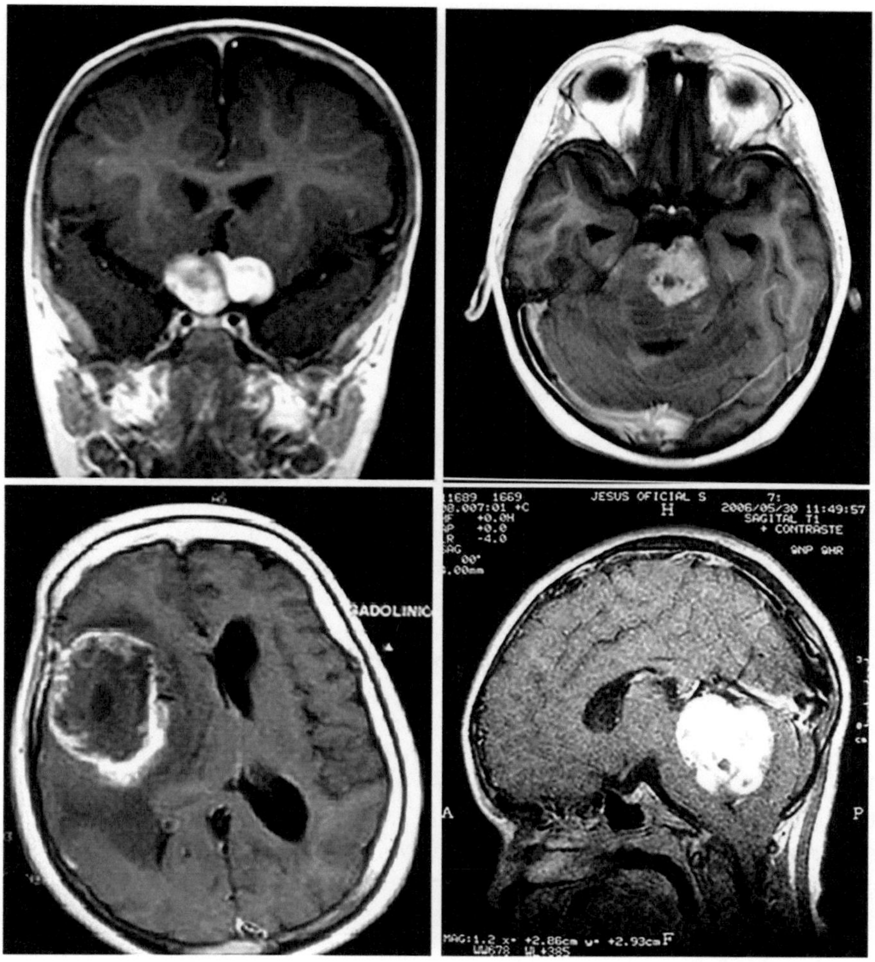

Figure 2.
(A and B) Pilocytic and diffuse astrocytoma. These tumors are both isodense and hypodense to the brain and show calcifications in 15–20% of cases, and they have virtually no edema. (C) Anaplastic astrocytoma is poorly defined lesions with heterogenous signal strengths. Mixed areas of isodensity to hipodensity are observed; these tumors may have hemorrhagic foci. It is common to observe a hypertensive central nucleus, which is surrounded by an intense edge with peripheral finger-like projections and secondary to a vasogenic edema. (D) GBM. Heterogenous lesion with cellular components of mixed signal, central necrosis, and hemorrhage; calcifications are rare.

Tumors that do not have any of these molecular tests—immunohistochemistry or sequencing—are subclassified as DAst-NOS or AAst-NOS, respectively [12].

2.2.1 Glioblastoma

According to the new WHO classification, the GBM was also classified into the group of diffuse gliomas and subclassified into the *IDH*-mutant or *IDH*-wildtype categories, or the NOS category. The *IDH*-wildtype form represents ~90% of cases and was associated with primary GBM (*de novo*), which are more common in patients older than 55 years of age [29]. Meanwhile, the *IDH*-mutant GBMs (~10%) are tumors that develop from low-grade diffuse glioma and are commonly present in younger patients; this type of GBM are also known as secondary GBM [29]. Similar to that described above, GBM-NOS are those tumors that do not have a full *IDH* evaluation [12]. According to phenotypic traits and the genetic background, to date, there are different GBM variants (**Table 1**).

2.3 Pediatric diffuse gliomas

Pediatric diffuse gliomas have the K27 mutation in the gene *H3F3A* (H3 Histone Family Member 3A) and less commonly in the related gene *HIST1H3B* (Histone Cluster 1 H3 Family Member B). Although they are mainly present in children, they can also be present in adults. These tumors exhibit a diffuse growth pattern and a midline location: thalamus, brain stem, and spinal cord; therefore, they are classified as diffuse midline glioma, H3 K27 mutant, and include tumors previously known as diffuse intrinsic pontine glioma (DIPG) [12].

3. LncRNAs in astrocytoma

LncRNAs have emerged as important molecular elements in different types of cancer, and Ast are not the exception [5, 30–32]. To date, diverse studies have shown the high complexity of the lncRNA study in Ast, due to the wide variety of mechanisms by which lncRNAs exerts their biological actions and because of the high tumor heterogeneity [33–35]. Changes in the nucleotide sequence of lncRNAs, their transcription rate, the expression of specific variants, in their expression levels, among others, could lead to an aberrant amplification of cell signals [36–38]. Given that GBM is the most aggressive type of cancer that begins within the brain [39, 40], most studies have been focused on this tumor subtype and to a lesser extent in the other WHO grades of adult Ast or in all WHO grades of p-Ast. Despite the significant effort that has been made in recent years to learn more about Ast, to the best of our knowledge, to date, there are very few molecular tools really applicable to diagnose, prognose, or treatment of these tumors [41–43]. Therefore, there is great interest to establish these molecular tools for GBM and evidence indicates that lncRNAs seem to be good candidates to serve such purpose.

3.1 LncRNAs as potential astrocytoma biomarkers

Expression changes of a biomolecule are a powerful tool to establish molecular "signatures" or "fingerprints" useful to distinguish and identify subgroups of a disease with a particular clinical behavior [44–47]. In this sense, expression changes of lncRNAs have been useful to differentiate both adult and pediatric Ast from nonneoplastic tissues, and some of them have the potential to be used in the medical practice as biomarkers. The meta-analysis performed by Zhang et al. [48] demonstrated for the first time the usefulness of the lncRNAs aberrantly expressed for Ast diagnosis and prognosis. This study showed that the expression profile of lncRNAs allowed to differentiate Ast or oligodendrogliomas from nonneoplastic tissues and to associate it with Ast malignancy or with lineage distinction in gliomas (**Table 2**). Subsequently, the same group established the first "molecular signature" of lncRNAs for Ast diagnosis and prognosis, which distinguished this neoplasia from nonneoplastic tissues, as well as Ast malignancy or patient's survival (**Table 2**) [49]. Additionally, a second group of precise lncRNAs was specific for Ast, and it was functional to differentiate them from the control tissues; from this signature, two lncRNAs were also associated with Ast malignancy, since their expression distinguished Ast WHO grades (**Table 2**) [50]. However, none of the lncRNAs that were part of the first molecular signature was established in the second, which could be related to the samples included in each study—referring to age, sex, with or without treatment, radiotherapy, among others—, as well as to the bioinformatic approach used in each study. This evidence emphasizes the importance that has the

Molecular signature (possible biomarkers for Ast diagnosis)	LncRNAs associated with Ast malignancy (possible biomarkers for Ast prognosis)	LncRNAs associated with patient's survival (possible biomarkers for prognosis)
Zhang et al. 2012; 2013		
KIAA0495 PART1 MGC21881 MIAT GAS5 PAR5 } Up-regulated	CRNDE-A CRNDE-B HOTAIRM1 } Up-regulated RP11-361F15.2-A RP11-361F15.2-B RFPL1S NCRNA00086 C21orf131-A } Down-regulated	KIAA0495 } Poor prognosis PART1 MGC21881 MIAT GAS5 PAR5 } Better prognosis
Zhi et al. 2015		
ENST00000244906 ENST00000545440 NR_002809 ENST00000436616 } Up-regulated XLOC_010967 BC002811 ASO1937 } Down-regulated	ENST00000545440 NR_002809	NR_002809 BC002811 XLOC_010967 } Poor prognosis
Matjasic et al. 2017		
LOC285758 } Up-regulated/ hypomethylated	LOC285758 gradual increase in its expression from grade I to GBM.	
Xu et al. 2017		
		lnc-C19orf57-6:6 lnc-ALYREF-1:1 SNHG1 } Poor prognosis

Table 2.
Molecular signatures of lncRNAs in astrocytoma.

homogenization of patient's samples included in a study has and how crucial it is to specify the clinic features of the included patients.

In addition to changes in the lncRNA expression, their promoter methylation status seems to be useful for Ast diagnosis and prognosis. Specifically, it was shown that expression and the promoter methylation pattern of *LOC285758* (Long Intergenic Non-Protein Coding RNA 1268) differentiate all Ast WHO grades and other gliomas (oligodendroglioma and oligoastrocitoma (II–III)) from the control, as well as Ast grades I–III from both primary and secondary GBM (**Table 2**) [32]. Based on this evidence, the identification of the mechanisms that lead to an aberrant expression of the lncRNAs—such as epigenetic regulation—could be part of the biomarkers package useful in the medical practice.

3.2 LncRNAs as potential GBM biomarkers

Specifically for GBM, different lncRNAs have also been found as potential biomarkers for its diagnosis and prognosis (**Table 3**). In this sense, Xu et al. [51] identified lncRNAs, which were associated with patient's survival; particularly, high expression of *SNHG1* (small nucleolar RNA host gene 1) was related with poor prognosis (**Table 3**). Meanwhile, *in silico* analysis showed many differentially expressed lncRNAs useful to distinguish GBM from nonneoplastic tissues and each

Diagnosis	CRNDE CYTOR	Up-regulated
	TUNAR LINCO1476	Down-regulated
Prognosis	CRNDE	Poor prognosis
	SNHG1	Poor prognosis
	RP11-334C17.6	High expression → Higher median survival times Low expression → Lower median survival times
	BTAT10	High expression → Lower median survival times Low expression Higher median survival times
	Circulating lncRNAs	
	HOTAIR GAS5	Up-regulated → Survival and GBM progression
	MALAT1	High expression: Poor overall survival; High recurrence of the disease
TMZ resistance	RP11-838N2.4 MALAT1 H19	Up-regulated

Table 3.
LncRNAs as potential GBM biomarkers.

of the four GBM subtypes: classical, mesenchymal, neural, and proneural. The lncRNAs *CRNDE* (colorectal neoplasia differentially expressed) and *CYTOR* (cytoskeleton regulator RNA) (both upregulated) and *TUNAR* (TCL1 upstream neural differentiation-associated RNA) and *LINCO1476* (both downregulated) were those with the highest expression changes in GBM compared to the control and with a potential use for GBM diagnosis (**Table 3**) [52]. *CRNDE* overexpression has been associated with high cell proliferation, migration, and invasion, which corresponds with the promotion of tumor growth observed in *in vivo* studies [53]. In addition, the expression pattern of *RP11-334C17.6* and *BTA10* allows to group patients with a greater survival from those with worse results, as well as the prognosis of each of the four GBM subtypes [52]. Currently, the available data are promising, and based on them, specific lncRNAs have been postulated as potential biomarkers for GBM diagnosis and prognosis, which with further evidence could be used in the medical practice.

3.3 Circulating lncRNAs

It is a fact that the establishment of novel biomarkers for Ast is essential and their identification and clinical application by means of less invasive methods would be ideal. To date, many studies have demonstrated the usefulness of circulating lncRNAs for diagnosis and prognosis of many diseases, including GBM [46, 54, 55]. The profile expression of lncRNAs was determined in blood serum of GBM patients and high levels of *HOTAIR* (HOX transcript antisense RNA) and *GAS5* [growth arrest specific 5 (nonprotein coding)] were prognostic factors to determine patient's survival and GBM progression [56]. Overexpression of circulating *HOTAIR* has been observed in different types of cancer [57–61], but its downregulation was detected in patients with acute myocardial infarction [62]. Interestingly, the presence of high levels of circulating *HOTAIR* DNA was also detected in breast cancer (BC) patients, where it has a potential use for BC diagnosis [60]. Unlike those observed in the GBM, most studies have shown that circulating *GAS5* was downexpressed in different types of cancer, which allowed the diagnosis of both intraductal papillary mucinous neoplasms [63] and nonsmall cell lung cancer [64, 65], as well as BC prognosis [66]. By contrast, overexpression of circulating GAS5 could be used to predict treatment response in head and neck cancer [67]. According to this, the overexpression of *HOTAIR* observed in all cancer types studied to date strongly suggests a central function of this lncRNA in the establishment, maintenance, and/or progression of cancer in general. Therefore, it is very important to identify the processes that *HOTAIR* is controlling in cancer in order to postulate molecular tools to eradicate neoplastic cells.

MALAT1 [metastasis associated lung adenocarcinoma transcript 1 (nonprotein coding)] was another lncRNA with changes on its circulating expression levels in GBM. This lncRNA was overexpressed, and this was associated with poor overall survival and with a high GBM recurrence [19]. Overexpression of circulating *MALAT1* has been observed in many types of cancer and it seems to be useful for cancer diagnosis and prognosis [68–73]. On the contrary, Peng et al. [74] showed that *MALAT1* downregulation in blood was important for early diagnosis in nonsmall cell lung cancer. Based on the above, the presence of a biomolecule in distinct corporal fluids is a noninvasive form at the molecular level either by the presence or the absence of a disease, as well as by the patient's prognosis with an specific disease. According to the studies performed to date, the use of circulating lncRNAs in the medical practice seems very promising.

3.4 Search for GBM biomarkers from a system biological perspective

Since a biomolecule does not act alone and depends on the cellular context to carry out its biological functions, different groups of study have focused on the identification of the lncRNA interactome in GBM. Evidence indicates that lncRNAs could interact with themselves, as well as with other biomolecules, such as mRNAs, miRNAs, and proteins; changes on the lncRNA activity at distinct molecular levels could affect their interaction networks and the correct cellular functioning [5, 75–77].

Yan et al. [78] established interaction networks between lncRNAs and mRNAs aberrantly expressed in GBM, and based on this, they postulated "hub genes" which were involved in GBM pathogenesis. Similarly, under this perspective, it was found that complexes conformed by lncRNA•mRNA (*HOTAIR-MX11-CD58/PRKCE* and *HOTAIR-ATF5-NCAM1*) or lncRNA•lncRNA (*MCM3AP-AS*-MIR17HG) could be potential biomarkers for GBM prognosis [79–82]. Importantly, the *TP73-AS1•RFX1* complex (TP73 Antisense RNA 1 and Regulatory Factor X1, respectively) was identified as an important factor for the control of apoptosis in this type of tumor [83]. To sum up, the cancer study from a system biological perspective has allowed to identify the complex interaction networks where many biomolecules are involved to regulate specific cellular processes; alterations in the operation of any of these components will affect the correct functioning of the cell. Specifically, lncRNA changes could lead to an amplification of the aberrant signals and this could be more significant if the lncRNAs interact with other ncRNAs, given that they have many targets of regulation.

3.5 Radio and chemoresistance

A major clinical problem is the resistance to chemotherapy and radiotherapy; therefore, identification of "molecular tools" that can predict and in the best-case scenario, improve the cellular response to these treatments would be ideal. Wang et al. [80] established a prediction model for radiosensitivity by detecting differential expressed lncRNAs and mRNAs after irradiation. Interestingly, the algorithm differentiated those patients that were radiosensitive and with a greater survival, from the patients with radioresistance; unfortunately, as far as we know, this is the only study focused on GBM radioresistance.

In addition, the involvement of lncRNAs in chemoresistance has been widely studied. LncRNAs *RP11-838 N2.4* [84] and *MALAT1* [19, 55] were shown to be associated with TMZ resistance (**Table 3**). Hiseq sequencing identified the profile expression of lncRNAs, which was specific and differentiated patient resistant to TMZ from those sensitive to this drug. This analysis showed that overexpression of *MALAT1* and its circulating form was related to a lower response to chemotherapy and to a shorter survival time of patients with GBM by controlling the miR-203 and *TYMS* (thymidylate synthase) levels, which was tested in TMZ resistant GBM cells [19]. Another fact worthy of mention is that other components of the *MALAT1* interactome have been elucidated to be important for TMZ resistance. *MALAT1* overexpression maintained high levels of expression of specific genes, such as *ABCB1* (ATP binding cassette subfamily B member 1), *ABCC5* (ATP binding cassette subfamily C member 5), *LRP1* (LDL receptor related protein 1), and *ZEB1* (zinc finger E-box binding homeobox). Notably, forced decrease of *MALAT1* resulted in TMZ sensitization by decreasing the levels of *ZEB1* [55]. Meanwhile, alterations in the axis RP11-838 N2.4•miR-10•EphA8 (EPH Receptor A8) were also involved in GBM cell resistance to TMZ [21]. All these facts supported the importance of the study of lncRNAs for clinical purposes and specifically gain knowledge regarding the prognosis of patients to radiotherapy or chemotherapy.

3.6 LncRNAs in stem cells

Many lines of evidence have shown the involvement of lncRNAs in the control of many cellular processes in cancer stem cells (CSCs) [85–87], but their participation in Ast has been very poorly studied. These cells are able to self-renew and differentiate into diverse cancer cell lineages to form tumors, so CSCs have been proposed as potential targets for cancer treatment. To further understand this, Balci et al. [88] determined the profile expression of lncRNAs in GBM stem cells (GSCs) relative to control stem cells. From these differentially expressed lncRNAs, *PCAT-1* (prostate cancer associated transcript 1 (nonprotein coding)), *MEG3* (maternally expressed 3 (nonprotein coding)), and *HOTAIR* functioned as tumor suppressors in GBM. This was related to alterations in gene expression. Interestingly, another study identified that even identical GSCs showed variations in their expression profile of lncRNAs, as well as in the variants produced by specific subgroups of cells. Despite this, the authors could establish a stem cell signature of 31 lncRNAs according to their expression levels [57]. Meanwhile, in hypoxic conditions, the expression of the lncRNA *HIF1A-AS2* (hypoxia inducible factor 1 alpha-antisense RNA 2) was induced and this led to positive control of the growth, self-renewal, and molecular reprograming of the GSCs [20]. Significantly, the control of these cellular processes was possible by regulating an interaction network, which will be described later.

Although many studies have focused on studying the changes on the expression of lncRNAs, very few have attempted to determine the mechanisms underlying this deregulation. In this sense, Zhang et al. [89] showed a feedback loop which controlled the expression of the lncRNA *FOXM1-AS* (Forkhead box M1 antisense) and it proved to be important for GSC tumorigenesis. *ALKBH5* (AlkB homolog 5, RNA demethylase) is a demethylase highly expressed in GBM GSCs, which was associated with an enhanced self-renewal and tumorigenesis of these cells. These malignant cell processes were controlled by *FOXM1* (Forkhead box M1) and *FOXM1-AS*, which increased their expression levels by a greater demethylation of the immature transcripts of *FOXM1*. In this pathway of regulation, *FOXM1-AS* was important to facilitate the action of *ALKBH5* on the nascent transcripts of *FOXM1*; therefore, a therapy in which the action of this lncRNA was reduced or blocked could be important to prevent GBM tumorigenesis. Taken together, these studies showed that although expression changes of lncRNAs were useful for GBM diagnosis and prognosis, they necessarily not represent the entire tumor, but rather this seems to associate with certain subgroups of cells that predominate over others and express particular lncRNAs. Therefore, the applicability of a differentially expressed biomolecule in the medical practice—particularly lncRNAs—must be done with caution and with all the required evidence.

4. Action mechanisms of lncRNAs in GBM

In addition to expression changes, it is necessary for the elucidation of the action mechanisms by which lncRNAs are acting. Evidence showed that lncRNAs act at both cytoplasmic and nuclear levels and that this is done directly and/or by their interaction with protein complexes and/or with other lncRNAs or different RNA species, such as mRNAs and miRNAs [5, 75–77]. Also, lncRNAs can regulate many signaling pathways by controlling the cytoplasmic disposal of mRNAs and miRNAs and even by producing small RNA species, such as miRNAs [89].

4.1 Sponge lncRNAs

This class of lncRNAs regulates miRNA disposal in the cell cytoplasm by capturing them and blocking their action [90, 91]. To date, all lncRNAs identified as "sponges" in the GBM acting as suppressors and involved in lncRNA upregulation and miRNA attenuation were associated with GBM **Table 4**). LncRNAs *H19* (imprinted maternally expressed transcript (nonprotein coding)) and *NEAT1* (nuclear paraspeckle assembly transcript 1 (nonprotein coding)) controlled the action of the miRNA let-7e, whose levels were downregulated in GBM due to the overexpression of these lncRNAs [92, 93]. Specifically, the axis *H19*•let-7e was involved in maintaining the phenotype of stem cells, which was associated with tumor malignancy and TMZ chemoresistance [93]. Similarly, a low disposal of let-7e by *NEAT1* overexpression, resulted in a higher activity of its mRNA target *NRAS* (NRAS proto-oncogene, GTPase), which leads to GBM malignancy [92].

"Sponges" LncRNAs	microRNA	mRNA target	Cellular process altered	Signaling pathway
Tumor suppressors				
H19 NEAT1	Let-7e	NRAS (NRAS Proto-Oncogene, GTPase)	H19: stem cells phenotype NEAT1:	
XIST	miR-152		Proliferation, migration, invasion, apoptosis evasion, tumor growth and poor mice survival	
TUG1	miR-299	VEGFA (Vascular Endothelial Growth Factor A)	Angiogenesis induction	
RP11-838N2.4	miR-10	EphA8 (EPH Receptor A8)	Apoptosis evasion	Apoptosis
SNHG7	miR-5095	CTNNB1 (Catenin Beta 1)	Proliferation, migration, invasion, apoptosis evasion	Wnt/β catenin
MALAT1	miR-203	TYMS (Thymidylate Synthetase)	Low chemotherapy response Shorter survival time of patients	
CRNDE	miR-136-5p	Wnt2 (Wnt Family Member A2) BCL2 (BCL2 Apoptosis Regulator)	Apoptosis evasion	Wnt Apoptosis
CASC2	miR-101	CPEB1 (Cytoplasmic Polyadenylation Element Binding Protein 1)	Cell proliferation Tumorigenesis	

Table 4.
LncRNAs as sponges in adult GBM.

Other lncRNAs that function as sponges in GBM were related to tumor malignancy. For example, the upregulation of *XIST* (X inactive specific transcript (nonprotein coding)) was related to GSC malignancy, tumor growth, and poor mice survival by controlling the action of miR-152 [94]. Meanwhile, the attenuation of the miR-299 disposal was controlled by the overexpression of *TUG1* (lncRNA taurine upregulated 1), which was related to tumor malignancy by the overactivation of *VEGFA* (vascular endothelial growth factor A) [95] and apoptosis evasion [93].

Similarly, GBM malignancy was mediated by the overexpression of *RP11-838N2.4* and *SNHG7* (small nucleolar RNA host gene 7), which regulated the function of miR-10 and miR-5095, respectively. In the first case, the attenuation of the action of miR-10 was associated with apoptosis evasion, and the reestablishment of the axis *RP11-838 N2.4*•miR-10•*EphA8* (EPH receptor A8) induced this programmed cell death [21]. Meanwhile, reestablishment of the *SNGH7*•miR-5095•*CTNNB1* (catenin beta 1) axis arrested tumor growth and decreased metastasis by decreasing the expression of *CTNNB1*, which is involved in the Wnt/β-catenin pathway [96]. Finally, it was observed that GBM proliferation, migration, and invasion were also promoted by the overexpression of *CRNDE* and the consequent attenuation of the miR-136-5p expression; all these led to the overactivation of BCL2 and WNT2, which are target genes of this miRNA [97]. According to the LNCipedia compendium, there are many variants reported for these lncRNAs; therefore, it would be very interesting and important to identify which lncRNA variants are expressed in GBM and which of them have the binding sites for trapping these miRNAs. Also, further studies are necessary to know if *H19* and *NEAT1* regulate the action of let-7e in a synergistic manner.

A very interesting case was that of the lncRNA *CASC2c* (cancer susceptibility candidate 2; formerly C10orf5). Besides its interaction with miR-101, this lncRNA was involved in the processing of the pre-miR-101 into mature miR-101 and competed with this miRNA for the mRNA *CPEB1* (cytoplasmic polyadenylation element binding protein 1). High levels of *CASC2c* and consequently a reduced activity of the axis miR-101•CPEB1 were associated with a high cell proliferation and tumorigenesis. Therefore, a decrease in *CASC2c* expression and an increased disposal of miR-101 were related to better patient's prognosis [98]. This evidence is an indication of all biological functions that an lncRNA can play in the cell and how the system ensures the regulation of gene expression by regulating at different levels the biogenesis of miRNAs (**Figure 3**). In consequence, if something modifies the processing of the pre-miR-101 or affects the regulation of its mature form, *CASC2c* would try to compensate the miRNA action by competing for its target genes. Evidently, other mechanisms must be involved in the biogenesis of this miRNA.

4.2 By interacting with mRNAs

Besides the lncRNA interaction with miRNAs, there is evidence indicating that lncRNAs can carry out their biological functions when they interact with mRNAs and/or proteins [5, 75–77]. As mentioned above, *HIF1A-AS2* was involved in the GSC malignancy under hypoxia conditions. The action of this lncRNA was performed in part by directly interacting with *IGF2BP2* (insulin-like growth factor 2 MRNA binding protein 2) and *DHX9* (DExH-box helicase 9), which finally controlled the action of *HMGA1* (high mobility group AT-Hook 1) [20]. According to this, elucidation of all the components that formed the interactome network of HIF1A-AS2 in the GSCs would be crucial to establish molecular tools for GBM treatment.

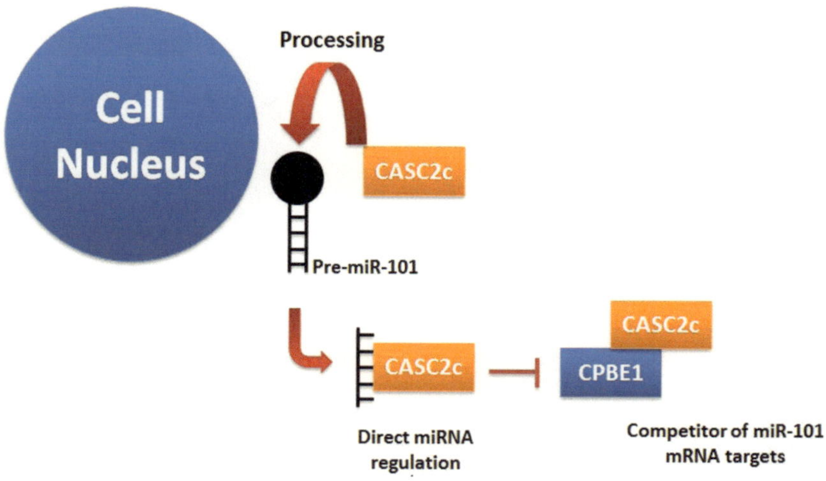

Figure 3.
The lncRNA CASC2 regulated the function of the miR-101 at different molecular levels. CASC2 was involved in the processing of the pre-miR-101 and also interact with its mature form to regulate the function of this miRNA. If any of these mechanisms fail, CASC2 ensures the miR-101 regulation by interacting with its mRNA targets.

5. Pediatric Ast

Adult and p-Ast are distinct molecular entities and are classified into different groups; therefore, studies in pediatric Ast are imperative. The first study performed in p-Ast was the one where the overexpression *HOTAIR* and *HOX* was detected in different pediatric brain tumors, including juvenile pediatric Ast (JPA); however, the biological meaning of this was not further studied [99].

We identified in the laboratory the expression profile of lncRNAs in p-Ast of WHO grades I–IV, given that the function of lncRNAs in p-Ast has been poorly studied. Similar to that observed for adult Ast, p-Ast showed many lncRNAs with expression changes relative to the control tissues, among histological grades or even in the same histological grade [5]. In addition, it was identified that the interaction of many differentially expressed lncRNAs with mRNAs and/or miRNAs aberrantly expressed was identified. As explained above, these interactions could lead to the amplification of the aberrant signals and to the modification of many signaling pathways. According to this, there were several hub lncRNAs in p-Ast that in relation to their interactions with mRNAs could be altering pathways such as FOXO, chemokine, hedgehog, MAPK, and others (**Figure 4**). Additionally, hub lncRNAs potentially useful to distinguish GBM from the other histopathological WHO grades were predicted to control diverse metabolic pathways and signaling pathways such as Ras, hippo, apellin, etc. (**Figure 4**).

The interaction of differentially expressed lncRNAs and miRNAs was shown to be a complex network that could be involved in modifications on proteoglycans in cancer, fatty acid metabolism, cell cycle, and spliceosome. Notably, data analysis revealed the presence of circular lncRNAs (circRNAs) with expression changes in p-Ast (**Figure 5**). According to the interactions of circRNAs with miRNAs, this type

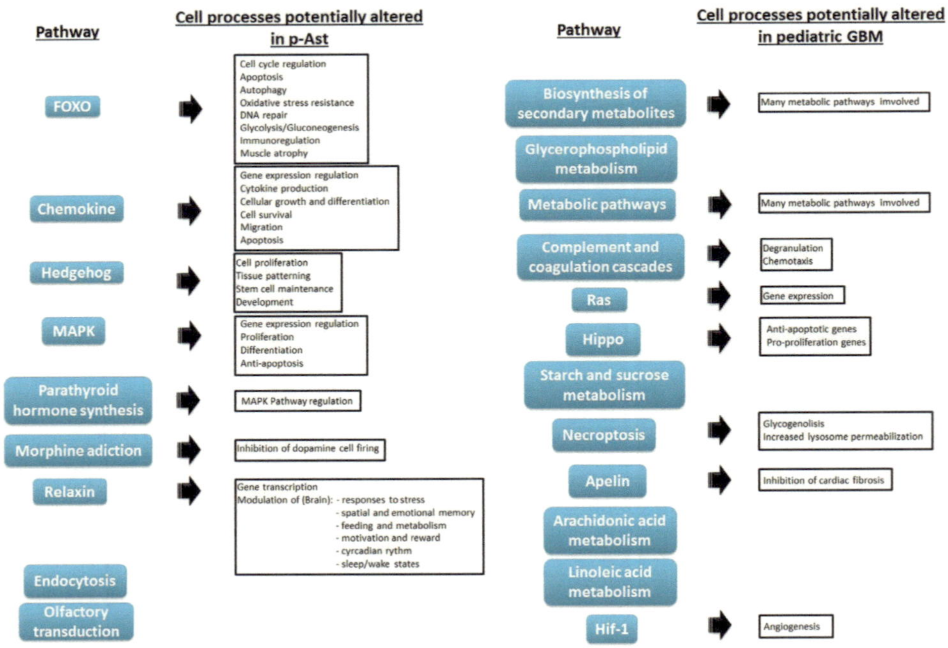

Figure 4.
Predicted interaction networks between lncRNAs and mRNAs were predicted to be involved in the control of signaling pathways. Data showed hub mRNAs that were analyzed with the KEGG (Kyoto Encyclopedia of Genes and Genomes) database. Hub mRNAs were those mRNAs with the highest number of interactions with lncRNAs. Data were taken from [5] and analyzed with KEGG.

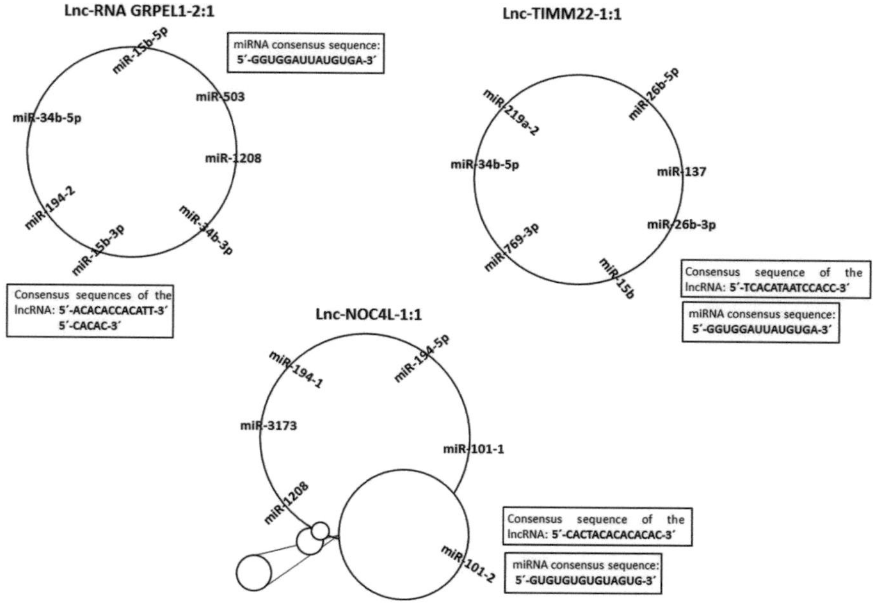

Figure 5.
Circular lncRNAs in pediatric astrocytoma. Predictions showed differentially expressed circRNAs in pediatric astrocytoma, which have many binding sites for miRNAs.

of lncRNAs was predicted to be involved in regulating cellular growth, survival, migration, invasion, adhesion, among others [5] (**Table 5**).

The integration of proteome and mirnome, as well as transcriptome data showed a convergence of all these biomolecules in the control of common signaling pathways, which gave an overview of the action of complex networks in cancer, particularly p-Ast [5, 47]. For example, although it is widely known that the MAPK pathway is altered in ~88% of gliomas, these data showed novel molecular components involved in this signaling pathway in p-Ast, which also allow to differentiate GBM from the other histological grades. The lncRNA *GRPEL1-1:1* was aberrantly expressed in all p-Ast grades when compared to the control tissues, but it was downregulated in WHO grades I–III relative to GBM. It is noteworthy to add, this lncRNA was predicted to interact with miR-15b-5p, and its expression levels were inversely correlated to those of *lnc-GRPEL1-1:1* (**Figure 6**). Other lncRNAs such as *TIMM22-1:1*, *Noc4L-1:1*, and *LINC-ROR* were predicted to be involved in the MAPK pathway, as well as in the Wnt pathway and extracellular matrix interactions [5]. In pediatric GBM, the overexpression of linc-Ror could lead to the downregulation of miR-145, since there is evidence indicating that linc-Ror sponges to miR-145, which was associated with cancer malignancy [100, 101]. According to our model, the linc-Ror•miR-145 axis could be increasing the expression of *IGFR1* (insulin-like growth factor 1 receptor), *c-Myc* (MYC proto-oncogene, BHLH transcription factor), and *STAT1* (signal transducer and activator of transcription 1), which causes a sustained angiogenesis and increased cell proliferation; however, this must be tested (**Figure 6**). In patients with glioma, linc-Ror was downregulated and this correlated positively and negatively with the expression of *SOX11* (SRY-box 11) and *KFL4* (Kruppel-like factor 4), respectively [101]. In the GBM cell line U87, *in vitro* assays showed the involvement of this lncRNA in the induction of cell proliferation, *CD133* expression, and in the formation of neurospheres [101], which are the factors of tumor malignancy. Similarly, linc-Ror was downregulated in p-Ast grades I–III, but it was upregulated in GBM relative to control tissues and other p-Ast grades [5]. Therefore, linc-Ror seems to be a candidate to function as a biomarker for p-Ast diagnosis and prognosis.

KEGG pathway	p-value	Number of genes	Number of miRNAs	Potential cellular processes altered
Proteoglycans in cancer	8.91e−11	120	14	Cellular growth and survival Cell migration and invasion Cell adhesion Apoptosis Angiogenesis Vascular permeability
Fatty acid metabolism	9.64e−09	28	12	Fatty acid metabolism
Adherens junction	3.85e−08	49	12	Actin polymerization Cell growth and differentiation Gene expression
Cell cycle	3.85e−08	85	14	Ubiquitin mediated proteolysis DNA biosynthesis Origin recognition complex Mini-Chromosome maintenance
Protein processing in the endoplasmic reticulum	2.59e−07	101	14	Proteasome Apoptosis
Fatty acid elongation	1.78e-06	13	7	Fatty acid degradation Fatty acid biosynthesis
p53 signaling pathway	2.12e−06	50	14	Cell cycle arrest Apoptosis Inhibition of angiogenesis and metastasis DNA repair and damage prevention Inhibition of IGF-1/mTOR pathway Exosome mediated secretion p53 negative feedback Cellular senescence
Hippo signaling pathway	2.29e-06	77	14	Pro-apoptotic genes Anti-apoptotic genes Pro-proliferation genes Cell contact inhibition Organ size control Adherens junctions
TGF-beta signaling pathway	2.32e−06	48	12	Differentiation, neurogenesis, ventral mesoderm specification Angiogenesis, extracellular matrix neogenesis, immunosuppression, apoptosis induction. G1 arrest Gonadal growth, embryo differentiation, placenta formation Left-right axis determination
Prion diseases	9.44e−06	15	9	Neuronal apoptosis Autophagy Oxidative stress Proliferation of astrocytes

Table 5.
Pathways potentially regulated by differentially expressed super sponges in pediatric astrocytoma; DIANA MirPath V 3.0 analysis.

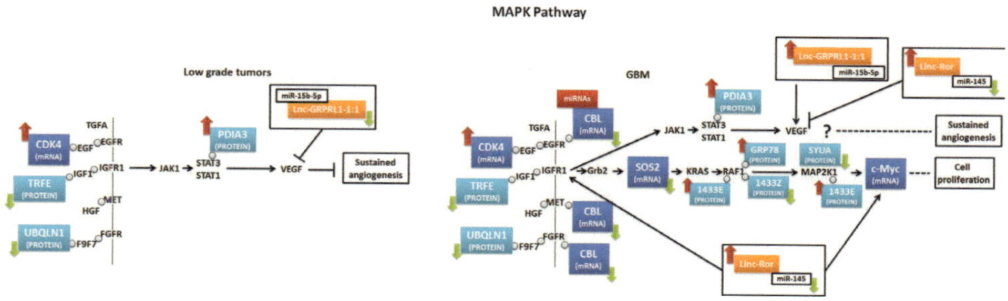

Figure 6.
LncRNAs were predicted to be involved in the control of signaling pathways. Differentially expressed lncRNAs were involved in controlling many signaling pathways by interacting with both mRNAs and miRNAs. Further experimental validation is necessary.

6. Conclusions

The lncRNA study in Ast has demonstrated an aberrant expression of this type of RNAs in both tumors and blood, which was useful to distinguish Ast from its nonneoplastic counterpart. The elucidation of molecular signatures from circulating lncRNAs is very promising due to their potential use as noninvasive tools for the diagnosis and prognosis of Ast. From another approach, it could be relevant the identification of complete interaction networks in which lncRNAs, other RNA species, and proteins were involved, since this would give a "panoramic vision" of how the aberrant system functions in astrocytic tumors. This could be crucial for the creation of molecular tools for their treatment.

Acknowledgements

This work was partially supported by the grant FIS/IMSS/PROT/G17 from The Mexican Institute of Social Security (IMSS). The English edition was carried out by Areli Ruiz Esparza, translator in-chief at SINTAGMA TRANSLATIONS.

Conflict of interest

All the authors declare that there is no conflict of interest.

Author details

Ruth Ruiz Esparza-Garrido[1], Alicia Siordia-Reyes[2], Gerardo Sánchez[3], Griselda Ramírez[3] and Miguel Velázquez-Flores[1*]

1 Functional Genomics Laboratory, Unit of Medical Research on Human Genomics, Children's Hospital "Silvestre Frenk Freund", National Medical Center Century XXI, Institute of Social Security (IMSS), CDMX, Mexico

2 Pediatric Pathology Service, Children's Hospital "Silvestre Frenk Freund", National Medical Center Century XXI, Institute of Social Security (IMSS), CDMX, Mexico

3 Pediatric Neurosurgery Service, Children's Hospital "Silvestre Frenk Freund", National Medical Center Century XXI, Institute of Social Security (IMSS), CDMX, Mexico

*Address all correspondence to: dr.velazquez.imss@gmail.com

IntechOpen

© 2018 The Author(s). Licensee IntechOpen. This chapter is distributed under the terms of the Creative Commons Attribution License (http://creativecommons.org/licenses/by/3.0), which permits unrestricted use, distribution, and reproduction in any medium, provided the original work is properly cited.

References

[1] ENCODE Project Consortium. An integrated encyclopedia of DNA elements in the human genome. Nature. 2012;**489**:57-74. DOI: 10.1038/nature11247

[2] Zhang C, Zhao LM, Wu H, Tian G, Dai SL, Zhao RY, et al. C/D-Box Snord105b promotes tumorigenesis in gastric cancer via ALDOA/C-Myc pathway. Cellular Physiology and Biochemistry. 2018;**45**:2471-2482. DOI: 10.1159/000488265

[3] López-Aguilar JE, Velázquez-Flores MA, Simón-Martínez LA, Ávila-Miranda R, Rodríguez-Florido MA, Ruiz-Esparza Garrido R. Circulating microRNAs as biomarkers for pediatric astrocytomas. Archives of Medical Research. 2017;**48**:323-332. DOI: 10.1016/j.arcmed.2017.07.002

[4] Marshall EA, Sage AP, Ng KW, Martinez VD, Firmino NS, Bennewith KL, et al. Small non-coding RNA transcriptome of the NCI-60 cell line panel. Scientific Data. 2017;**4**:170157. DOI: 10.1038/sdata.2017.157

[5] Ruiz Esparza-Garrido R, Rodríguez-Corona JM, López-Aguilar JE, Rodríguez-Florido MA, Velázquez-Wong AC, Viedma-Rodríguez R, et al. Differentially expressed long non-coding RNAs were predicted to be involved in the control of signaling pathways in pediatric astrocytoma. Molecular Neurobiology. 2017;**54**:6598-6608. DOI: 10.1007/s12035-016-0123-9

[6] Jarroux J, Morillon A, Pinskaya M. History, discovery, and classification of lncRNAs. Advances in Experimental Medicine and Biology. 2017;**1008**:1-46. DOI: 10.1007/978-981-10-5203-3_1

[7] Necsulea A, Soumillon M, Warnefors M, Liechti A, Daish T, Zeller U, et al. The evolution of lncRNA repertoires and expression patterns in tetrapods. Nature. 2014;**505**:635-640. DOI: 10.1038/nature12943

[8] Botti G, Marra L, Malzone MG, Anniciello A, Botti C, Franco R, et al. LncRNA HOTAIR as prognostic circulating marker and potential therapeutic target in patients with tumor diseases. Current Drug Targets. 2017;**18**:27-34

[9] Noh JH, Kim KM, McClusky WG, Abdelmohsen K, Gorospe M. Cytoplasmic functions of long noncoding RNAs. Wiley Interdisciplinary Reviews: RNA. 2018;**9**:e1471. DOI: 10.1002/wrna.1471

[10] Ostrom QT, Gittleman H, Stetson L, Virk S, Barnholtz-Sloan JS. Epidemiology of intracranial gliomas. Progress in Neurological Surgery. 2018;**30**:1-11. DOI: 10.1159/000464374

[11] Ostrom QT, Gittleman H, Liao P, Rouse C, Chen Y, Dowling J, et al. CBTRUS statistical report: Primary brain and central nervous system tumors diagnosed in the United States in 2007-2011. Neuro-Oncology. 2014;**16**(Suppl 4):iv1-iv63

[12] Louis DN, Perry A, Reifenberger G, von Deimling A, Figarella-Branger D, Cavenee WK, et al. The 2016 World Health Organization classification of tumors of the central nervous system: A summary. Acta Neuropathologica. 2016;**131**:803-820. DOI: 10.1007/s00401-016-1545-1

[13] Kim W, Liau LM. IDH mutations in human glioma. Neurosurgery Clinics of North America. 2012;**23**:471-480. DOI: 10.1016/j.nec.2012.04.009

[14] Pathak P, Jha P, Purkait S, Sharma V, Suri V, Sharma MC, et al. Altered

global histone-trimethylation code and H3F3A-ATRX mutation in pediatric GBM. Journal of Neuro-Oncology. 2015;**121**:489-497. DOI: 10.1007/s11060-014-1675-z6

[15] Wu G, Diaz AK, Paugh BS, Rankin SL, Ju B, Li Y, et al. The genomic landscape of diffuse intrinsic pontine glioma and pediatric non-brainstem high-grade glioma. Nature Genetics. 2014;**46**:444-450. DOI: 10.1038/ng.2938

[16] Schwartzentruber J, Korshunov A, Liu XY, Jones DT, Pfaff E, Jacob K, et al. Driver mutations in histone H3.3 and chromatin remodelling genes in paediatric glioblastoma. Nature. 2012;**482**:226-231. DOI: 10.1038/nature10833

[17] Faury D, Nantel A, Dunn SE, Guiot M, Haque T, Hauser P, et al. Molecular profiling identifies prognostic subgroups of pediatric glioblastoma and shows increased YB-1 expression in tumors. Journal of Clinical Oncology. 2007;**25**:1196-1208. DOI: 10.1200/JCO.2006.07.8626

[18] Zeng H, Xu N, Liu Y, Liu B, Yang Z, Fu Z, et al. Genomic profiling of long non-coding RNA and mRNA expression associated with acquired temozolomide resistance in glioblastoma cells. International Journal of Oncology. 2017;**51**:445-455. DOI: 10.3892/ijo.2017.4033

[19] Chen W, Xu XK, Li JL, Kong KK, Li H, Chen C, et al. MALAT1 is a prognostic factor in glioblastoma multiforme and induces chemoresistance to temozolomide through suppressing miR-203 and promoting thymidylate synthase expression. Oncotarget. 2017;**8**:22783-22799. DOI: 10.18632/oncotarget.15199

[20] Mineo M, Ricklefs F, Rooj AK, Lyons SM, Ivanov P, Ansari KI, et al. The long non-coding RNA HIF1A-AS2 facilitates the maintenance of mesenchymal glioblastoma stem-like cells in hypoxic niches. Cell Reports. 2016;**15**:2500-2509. DOI: 10.1016/j.celrep.2016.05.018

[21] Liu Y, Xu N, Liu B, Huang Y, Zeng H, Yang Z, et al. Long noncoding RNA RP11-838N2.4 enhances the cytotoxic effects of temozolomide by inhibiting the functions of miR-10a in glioblastoma cell lines. Oncotarget. 2016;**7**:43835-43851. DOI: 10.18632/oncotarget.9699

[22] Louis DN, Ohgaki H, Wiestler OD, Cavenee WK, Burger PC, Jouvet A, et al. The 2007 WHO classification of tumours of the central nervous system. Acta Neuropathologica. 2007;**114**:97-109. DOI: 10.1007/s00401-007-0243-4

[23] Bristol RE. Low-grade glia tumors: Are they all the same? Seminars in Pediatric Neurology. 2000;**16**:23-26

[24] Broniscer A, Baker JS, West NA, Fraser MM, Proko E, Kocak M, et al. Clinical and molecular characteristics of malignant transformation of low-grade glioma in children. Journal of Clinical Oncology. 2007;**25**:682-689

[25] Pascual-Castroviejo I, Pascual-Pascual SI, Viaño J, Velázquez-Fragua R, Carceller-Benito F, Gutiérrez-Molina M, et al. Cerebral hemisphere tumours in neurofibromatosis type 1 during childhood. Revista de Neurologia. 2010;**50**:453-457

[26] Pong WW, Gutmann DH. The ecology of brain tumors: Lessons learned from neurofibromatosis-1. Oncogene. 2011;**30**:1135-1146. DOI: 10.1038/onc.2010.519

[27] Cancer Genome Atlas Research Network, Brat DJ, Verhaak RG, Aldape

KD, Yung WK, Salama SR, et al. Comprehensive, integrative genomic analysis of diffuse lower-grade gliomas. The New England Journal of Medicine. 2005;**372**:2481-2498. DOI: 10.1056/NEJMoa1402121

[28] Reuss DE, Kratz A, Sahm F, Capper D, Schrimpf D, Koelsche C, et al. Adult IDH wild type astrocytomas biologically and clinically resolve into other tumor entities. Acta Neuropathologica. 2015;**130**(3):407-417. DOI: 10.1007/s00401-015-1454-8

[29] Ohgaki H, Kleihues P. The definition of primary and secondary glioblastoma. Clinical Cancer Research. 2013;**19**:764-772. DOI: 10.1158/1078-0432.CCR-12-3002

[30] Huang SK, Luo Q, Peng H, Li J, Zhao M, Wang J, et al. A panel of serum noncoding RNAs for the diagnosis and monitoring of response to therapy in patients with breast cancer. Medical Science Monitor. 2018;**24**:2476-2488

[31] Ma Y, Luo T, Dong D, Wu X, Wang Y. Characterization of long non-coding RNAs to reveal potential prognostic biomarkers in hepatocellular carcinoma. Gene. 2018;**663**:148-153. pii:S0378-1119(18)30427-X. DOI: 10.1016/j.gene.2018.04.053

[32] Matjasic A, Popovic M, Matos B, Glavac D. Expression of LOC285758, a potential long non-coding biomarker, is methylation-dependent and correlates with glioma malignancy grade. Radiology and Oncology. 2017;**51**:331-341. DOI: 10.1515/raon-2017-0004

[33] Nakajima N, Nobusawa S, Nakata S, Nakada M, Yamazaki T, Matsumura N, et al. BRAF V600E, TERT promoter mutations and CDKN2A/B homozygous deletions are frequent in epithelioid glioblastomas: A histological and molecular analysis focusing on intratumoral heterogeneity. Brain Pathology. 2017. DOI: 10.1111/bpa.12572

[34] Smith SJ, Diksin M, Chhaya S, Sairam S, Estevez-Cebrero MA, Rahman R. The invasive region of glioblastoma defined by 5ALA guided surgery has an altered cancer stem cell marker profile compared to central tumour. International Journal of Molecular Sciences. 2017;**18**:E2452. DOI: 10.3390/ijms18112452

[35] Hu W, Wang T, Yang Y, Zheng S. Tumor heterogeneity uncovered by dynamic expression of long noncoding RNA at single-cell resolution. Cancer Genetics. 2015;**208**:581-586. DOI: 10.1016/j.cancergen.2015.09.005

[36] Jiang Y, Du F, Chen F, Qin N, Jiang Z, Zhou J, et al. Potentially functional variants in lncRNAs are associated with breast cancer risk in a Chinese population. Molecular Carcinogenesis. 2017;**56**:2048-2057. DOI: 10.1002/mc.22659

[37] Sen R, Doose G, Stadler PF. Rare splice variants in long non-coding RNAs. Noncoding RNA. 2017;**3**:E23. DOI: 10.3390/ncrna3030023

[38] Wang Y, Li Z, Zheng S, Zhou Y, Zhao L, Ye H, et al. Expression profile of long non-coding RNAs in pancreatic cancer and their clinical significance as biomarkers. Oncotarget. 2015;**6**:35684-35698. DOI: 10.18632/oncotarget.5533

[39] Bleeker FE, Molenaar RJ, Leenstra S. Recent advances in the molecular understanding of glioblastoma. Journal of Neuro-Oncology. 2012;**108**:11-27. DOI: 10.1007/s11060-011-0793-0

[40] McNeill KA. Epidemiology of brain tumors. Neurologic Clinics. 2016;**34**:981-998. DOI: 10.1016/j.ncl.2016.06.014

[41] Omuro A, Beal K, McNeill K, Young RJ, Thomas A, Lin X, et al. Multicenter phase IB trial of carboxyamidotriazole orotate and temozolomide for recurrent and newly diagnosed glioblastoma and other anaplastic gliomas. Journal of Clinical Oncology. 2018. DOI: JCO2017769992. DOI: 10.1200/JCO.2017.76.9992

[42] Roberto GM, Paiva HH, Botelho de Souza LE, Pezuk JA, Vieira GM, Francisco de Oliveira H, et al. DTCM-glutarimide delays growth and radiosensitizes glioblastoma. Anti-Cancer Agents in Medicinal Chemistry. 2018;**18**:1. DOI: 10.2174/1871520618666180423105740

[43] Sousa F, Moura RP, Moreira E, Martins C, Sarmento B. Therapeutic monoclonal antibodies delivery for the glioblastoma treatment. Advances in Protein Chemistry and Structural Biology. 2018;**112**:61-80. DOI: 10.1016/bs.apcsb.2018.03.001

[44] Álvarez-Chaver P, De Chiara L, Martínez-Zorzano VS. Proteomic profiling for colorectal cancer biomarker discovery. Methods in Molecular Biology. 2018;**1765**:241-269. DOI: 10.1007/978-1-4939-7765-9_16

[45] Assmann TS, Recamonde-Mendoza M, Puñales M, Tschiedel B, Canani LH, Crispim D. MicroRNA expression profile in plasma from Type 1 diabetic patients: Case-control study and bioinformatic analysis. Diabetes Research and Clinical Practice. 2018;**141**:35-46. pii:S0168-8227(17)32036-3. DOI: 10.1016/j.diabres.2018.03.044

[46] Umu SU, Langseth H, Bucher-Johannessen C, Fromm B, Keller A, Meese E, et al. A comprehensive profile of circulating RNAs in human serum. RNA Biology. 2018;**15**:242-250. DOI: 10.1080/15476286.2017.1403003

[47] Ruiz Esparza-Garrido R, Velázquez-Flores MÁ, Diegopérez-Ramírez J, López-Aguilar E, Siordia-Reyes G, Hernández-Ortiz M, et al. A proteomic approach of pediatric astrocytomas: MiRNAs and network insight. Journal of Proteomics. 2013;**94**:162-175. DOI: 10.1016/j.jprot.2013.09.009

[48] Zhang X, Sun S, Pu JK, Tsang AC, Lee D, Man VO, et al. Long non-coding RNA expression profiles predict clinical phenotypes in glioma. Neurobiology of Disease. 2012;**48**:1-8. DOI: 10.1016/j.nbd.2012.06.004

[49] Zhang XQ, Sun S, Lam KF, Kiang KM, Pu JK, Ho AS, et al. A long non-coding RNA signature in glioblastoma multiforme predicts survival. Neurobiology of Disease. 2013;**58**:123-131. DOI: 10.1016/j.nbd.2013.05.011

[50] Zhi F, Wang Q, Xue L, Shao N, Wang R, Deng D, et al. The use of three long non-coding RNAs as potential prognostic indicators of astrocytoma. PLoS One. 2015;**10**:e0135242. DOI: 10.1371/journal.pone.0135242

[51] Xu C, Qi R, Ping Y, Li J, Zhao H, Wang L, et al. Systemically identifying and prioritizing risk lncRNAs through integration of pan-cancer phenotype associations. Oncotarget. 2017;**8**(7):12041-12051. DOI: 10.18632/oncotarget.14510

[52] Reon BJ, Anaya J, Zhang Y, Mandell J, Purow B, Abounader R, et al. Expression of lncRNAs in low-grade gliomas and glioblastoma multiforme: An in silico analysis. PLoS Medicine. 2016;**13**:e1002192. DOI: 10.1371/journal.pmed.1002192

[53] Wang Y, Wang Y, Li J, Zhang Y, Yin H, Han B. CRNDE, a long-noncoding RNA, promotes glioma cell growth and invasion through mTOR signaling. Cancer Letters. 2015;**367**:122-128. DOI: 10.1016/j.canlet.2015.03.027

[54] Wang YH, Ji J, Wang BC, Chen H, Yang ZH, Wang K, et al. Tumor-derived exosomal long noncoding RNAs as promising diagnostic biomarkers for prostate cancer. Cellular Physiology and Biochemistry. 2018;**46**:532-545. DOI: 10.1159/000488620

[55] Li H, Yuan X, Yan D, Li D, Guan F, Dong Y, et al. Long non-coding RNA MALAT1 decreases the sensitivity of resistant glioblastoma cell lines to temozolomide. Cellular Physiology and Biochemistry. 2017;**42**:1192-1201. DOI: 10.1159/000478917

[56] Shen J, Hodges TR, Song R, Gong Y, Calin GA, Heimberger AB, et al. Serum HOTAIR and GAS5 levels as predictors of survival in patients with glioblastoma. Molecular Carcinogenesis. 2018;**57**:137-141. DOI: 10.1002/mc.22739

[57] Lv R, Zhang J, Zhang W, Huang Y, Wang N, Zhang Q, et al. Circulating HOTAIR expression predicts the clinical response to neoadjuvant chemotherapy in patients with breast cancer. Cancer Biomarkers. 2018;**22**:249-256. DOI: 10.3233/CBM-170874

[58] Cantile M, Scognamiglio G, Marra L, Aquino G, Botti C, Falcone MR, et al. HOTAIR role in melanoma progression and its identification in the blood of patients with advanced disease. Journal of Cellular Physiology. 2017;**232**: 3422-3432. DOI: 10.1002/jcp.25789

[59] Li N, Wang Y, Liu X, Luo P, Jing W, Zhu M, et al. Identification of circulating long noncoding RNA HOTAIR as a novel biomarker for diagnosis and monitoring of non-small cell lung cancer. Technology in Cancer Research & Treatment. 2017;**16**:1060-1066. DOI: 10.1177/1533034617723754

[60] Zhang L, Song X, Wang X, Xie Y, Wang Z, Xu Y, et al. Circulating DNA of HOTAIR in serum is a novel biomarker for breast cancer. Breast Cancer Research and Treatment. 2015;**152**:199-208. DOI: 10.1007/s10549-015-3431-2

[61] Li J, Wang Y, Yu J, Dong R, Qiu H. A high level of circulating HOTAIR is associated with progression and poor prognosis of cervical cancer. Tumour Biology. 2015;**36**:1661-1665. DOI: 10.1007/s13277-014-2765-4

[62] Gao L, Liu Y, Guo S, Yao R, Wu L, Xiao L, et al. Circulating long noncoding RNA HOTAIR is an essential mediator of acute myocardial infarction. Cellular Physiology and Biochemistry. 2017;**44**:1497-1508. DOI: 10.1159/000485588

[63] Permuth JB, Chen DT, Yoder SJ, Li J, Smith AT, Choi JW, et al. Linking circulating long non-coding RNAs to the diagnosis and malignant prediction of intraductal papillary mucinous neoplasms of the pancreas. Scientific Reports. 2017;**7**:10484. DOI: 10.1038/s41598-017-09754-5

[64] Tan Q, Zuo J, Qiu S, Yu Y, Zhou H, Li N, et al. Identification of circulating long non-coding RNA GAS5 as a potential biomarker for non-small cell lung cancer diagnosisnon-small cell lung cancer, long non-coding RNA, plasma, GAS5, biomarker. International Journal of Oncology. 2017;**50**:1729-1738. DOI: 10.3892/ijo.2017.3925

[65] Liang W, Lv T, Shi X, Liu H, Zhu Q, Zeng J, et al. Circulating long noncoding RNA GAS5 is a novel biomarker for the diagnosis of nonsmall cell lung cancer. Medicine (Baltimore). 2016;**95**:e4608. DOI: 10.1097/MD.0000000000004608

[66] Han L, Ma P, Liu SM, Zhou X. Circulating long noncoding RNA GAS5 as a potential biomarker in breast cancer for assessing the surgical effects. Tumour Biology. 2016;**37**:6847-6854. DOI: 10.1007/s13277-015-4568-7

[67] Fayda M, Isin M, Tambas M, Guveli M, Meral R, Altun M, et al. Do

circulating long non-coding RNAs (lncRNAs) (LincRNA-p21, GAS 5, HOTAIR) predict the treatment response in patients with head and neck cancer treated with chemoradiotherapy? Tumour Biology. 2016;**37**:3969-3978. DOI: 10.1007/s13277-015-4189-1

[68] Zidan HE, Karam RA, El-Seifi OS, Abd Elrahman TM. Circulating long non-coding RNA MALAT1 expression as molecular biomarker in Egyptian patients with breast cancer. Cancer Genetics. 2018;**220**:32-37. DOI: 10.1016/j.cancergen.2017.11.005

[69] Zhang R, Xia Y, Wang Z, Zheng J, Chen Y, Li X, et al. Serum long non coding RNA MALAT-1 protected by exosomes is up-regulated and promotes cell proliferation and migration in non-small cell lung cancer. Biochemical and Biophysical Research Communications. 2017;**490**(2):406-414. DOI: 10.1016/j.bbrc.2017.06.055

[70] He B, Zeng J, Chao W, Chen X, Huang Y, Deng K, et al. Serum long non-coding RNAs MALAT1, AFAP1-AS1 and AL359062 as diagnostic and prognostic biomarkers for nasopharyngeal carcinoma. Oncotarget. 2017;**8**:41166-41177. DOI: 10.18632/oncotarget.17083

[71] Duan W, Du L, Jiang X, Wang R, Yan S, Xie Y, et al. Identification of a serum circulating lncRNA panel for the diagnosis and recurrence prediction of bladder cancer. Oncotarget. 2016;7:78850-78858. DOI: 10.18632/oncotarget.12880

[72] Pang EJ, Yang R, Fu XB, Liu YF. Overexpression of long non-coding RNA MALAT1 is correlated with clinical progression and unfavorable prognosis in pancreatic cancer. Tumour Biology. 2015;**36**:2403-2407. DOI: 10.1007/s13277-014-2850-8

[73] Ren S, Liu Y, Xu W, Sun Y, Lu J, Wang F, et al. Long noncoding RNA MALAT-1 is a new potential therapeutic target for castration resistant prostate cancer. The Journal of Urology. 2013;**190**:2278-2287. DOI: 10.1016/j.juro.2013.07.001

[74] Peng H, Wang J, Li J, Zhao M, Huang SK, Gu YY, et al. A circulating non-coding RNA panel as an early detection predictor of non-small cell lung cancer. Life Sciences. 2016;**151**:235-242. DOI: 10.1016/j.lfs.2016.03.002

[75] Jalali S, Gandhi S, Scaria V. Distinct and modular organization of protein interacting sites in long non-coding RNAs. Frontiers in Molecular Biosciences. 2018;**5**:27. DOI: 10.3389/fmolb.2018.00027

[76] Li G, Liu K, Du X. Long non-coding RNA TUG1 promotes proliferation and inhibits apoptosis of osteosarcoma cells by sponging miR-132-3p and upregulating SOX4 expression. Yonsei Medical Journal. 2018;**59**:226-235. DOI: 10.3349/ymj.2018.59.2.226

[77] Sun XJ, Wang Q, Guo B, Liu XY, Wang B. Identification of skin-related lncRNAs as potential biomarkers that involved in Wnt pathways in keloids. Oncotarget. 2017;**8**:34236-34244. DOI: 10.18632/oncotarget.15880

[78] Yan Y, Zhang L, Jiang Y, Xu T, Mei Q, Wang H, et al. LncRNA and mRNA interaction study based on transcriptome profiles reveals potential core genes in the pathogenesis of human glioblastoma multiforme. Journal of Cancer Research and Clinical Oncology. 2015;**141**:827-838. DOI: 10.1007/s00432-014-1861-6

[79] Wang JB, Liu FH, Chen JH, Ge HT, Mu LY, Bao HB, et al. Identifying survival-associated modules from the dysregulated triplet network in glioblastoma multiforme. Journal of Cancer Research and Clinical Oncology. 2017;**143**:661-671. DOI: 10.1007/s00432-016-2332-z

[80] Cao Y, Wang P, Ning S, Xiao W, Xiao B, Li X. Identification of prognostic biomarkers in glioblastoma using a long non-coding RNA-mediated, competitive endogenous RNA network. Oncotarget. 2016;7:41737-41747. DOI: 10.18632/oncotarget.9569

[81] Li Q, Jia H, Li H, Dong C, Wang Y, Zou Z. LncRNA and mRNA expression profiles of glioblastoma multiforme (GBM) reveal the potential roles of lncRNAs in GBM pathogenesis. Tumour Biology. 2016;**37**:14537-14552

[82] Zhang K, Li Q, Kang X, Wang Y, Wang S. Identification and functional characterization of lncRNAs acting as ceRNA involved in the malignant progression of glioblastoma multiforme. Oncology Reports. 2016;**36**:2911-2925. DOI: 10.3892/or.2016.5070

[83] Wang WA, Lai LC, Tsai MH, Lu TP, Chuang EY. Development of a prediction model for radiosensitivity using the expression values of genes and long non-coding RNAs. Oncotarget. 2016;7:26739-26750. DOI: 10.18632/oncotarget.8496

[84] Izuogu OG, Alhasan AA, Mellough C, Collin J, Gallon R, Hyslop J, et al. Analysis of human ES cell differentiation establishes that the dominant isoforms of the lncRNAs RMST and FIRRE are circular. BMC Genomics. 2018;**19**:276. DOI: 10.1186/s12864-018-4660-7

[85] Ruan ZB, Chen GC, Ren Y, Zhu L. Expression profile of long non-coding RNAs during the differentiation of human umbilical cord derived mesenchymal stem cells into cardiomyocyte-like cells. Cytotechnology. 2018;**70**:1247-1260. DOI: 10.1007/s10616-018-0217-5

[86] Balci T, Yilmaz Susluer S, Kayabasi C, Ozmen Yelken B, Biray Avci C, Gunduz C. Analysis of dysregulated long non-coding RNA expressions in glioblastoma cells. Gene. 2016;**590**: 120-122. DOI: 10.1016/j.gene.2016.06.024

[87] Zhang S, Zhao BS, Zhou A, Lin K, Zheng S, Lu Z, et al. m6A demethylase ALKBH5 maintains tumorigenicity of glioblastoma stem-like cells by sustaining FOXM1 expression and cell proliferation program. Cancer Cell. 2017;**31**:591-606.e6. DOI: 10.1016/j.ccell.2017.02.013

[88] Ma X, Shao C, Jin Y, Wang H, Meng Y. Long non-coding RNAs: A novel endogenous source for the generation of Dicer-like 1-dependent small RNAs in Arabidopsis thaliana. RNA Biology. 2014;**11**:373-390. DOI: 10.4161/rna.28725

[89] Gaiti F, Hatleberg WL, Tanurdžić M, Degnan BM. Sponge long non-coding RNAs are expressed in specific cell types and conserved networks. Noncoding RNA. 2018;**4**:E6. DOI: 10.3390/ncrna4010006

[90] Zhou Y, Meng X, Chen S, Li W, Li D, Singer R, et al. IMP1 regulates UCA1-mediated cell invasion through facilitating UCA1 decay and decreasing the sponge effect of UCA1 for miR-122-5p. Breast Cancer Research. 2018;**20**:32. DOI: 10.1186/s13058-018-0959-1

[91] Gong W, Zheng J, Liu X, Ma J, Liu Y, Xue Y. Knockdown of NEAT1 restrained the malignant progression of glioma stem cells by activating microRNA let-7e. Oncotarget. 2016;**7**:62208-62223. DOI: 10.18632/oncotarget.11403

[92] Li W, Jiang P, Sun X, Xu S, Ma X, Zhan R. Suppressing H19 modulates tumorigenicity and stemness in U251 and U87MG glioma cells. Cellular and Molecular Neurobiology. 2016;**36**(8):1219-1227

[93] Yao Y, Ma J, Xue Y, Wang P, Li Z, Liu J, et al. Knockdown of long non-coding

RNA XIST exerts tumor-suppressive functions in human glioblastoma stem cells by up-regulating miR-152. Cancer Letters. 2015;**359**:75-86. DOI: 10.1016/j.canlet.2014.12.051

[94] Cai H, Liu X, Zheng J, Xue Y, Ma J, Li Z, et al. Long non-coding RNA taurine upregulated 1 enhances tumor-induced angiogenesis through inhibiting microRNA-299 in human glioblastoma. Oncogene. 2017;**36**:318-331. DOI: 10.1038/onc.2016.212

[95] Ren J, Yang Y, Xue J, Xi Z, Hu L, Pan SJ, et al. Long noncoding RNA SNHG7 promotes the progression and growth of glioblastoma via inhibition of miR-5095. Biochemical and Biophysical Research Communications. 2018;**496**:712-718. DOI: 10.1016/j.bbrc.2018.01.109

[96] Li DX, Fei XR, Dong YF, Cheng CD, Yang Y, Deng XF, et al. The long non-coding RNA CRNDE acts as a ceRNA and promotes glioma malignancy by preventing miR-136-5p-mediated downregulation of Bcl-2 and Wnt2. Oncotarget. 2017;**8**:88163-88178. DOI: 10.18632/oncotarget.21513

[97] Liu C, Sun Y, She X, Tu C, Cheng X, Wang L, et al. CASC2c as an unfavorable prognosis factor interacts with miR-101 to mediate astrocytoma tumorigenesis. Cell Death & Disease. 2017;**8**:e2639. DOI: 10.1038/cddis.2017.11

[98] Chakravadhanula M, Ozols VV, Hampton CN, Zhou L, Catchpoole D, Bhardwaj RD. Expression of the HOX genes and HOTAIR in a typical teratoid rhabdoid tumors and other pediatric brain tumors. Cancer Genetics. 2014;**207**:425-428. DOI: 10.1016/j.cancergen.2014.05.014

[99] Yan ZY, Sun XC. LincRNA-ROR functions as a ceRNA to regulate Oct4, Sox2, and Nanog expression by sponging miR-145 and its effect on biologic characteristics of colonic cancer stem cells. Zhonghua Bing Li Xue Za Zhi. 2018;**47**:284-290. DOI: 10.3760/cma.j.issn.0529-5807.2018.04.011

[100] Li C, Lu L, Feng B, Zhang K, Han S, Hou D, et al. The lincRNA-ROR/miR-145 axis promotes invasion and metastasis in hepatocellular carcinoma via induction of epithelial-mesenchymal transition by targeting ZEB2. Scientific Reports. 2017;**7**:4637. DOI: 10.1038/s41598-017-04113-w

[101] Feng S, Yao J, Chen Y, Geng P, Zhang H, Ma X, et al. Expression and functional role of reprogramming-related long noncoding RNA (lincRNA-ROR) in glioma. Journal of Molecular Neuroscience. 2015;**56**:623-630. DOI: 10.1007/s12031-014-0488-z

Chapter 4

Neurosurgical Tools to Improve Safety and Survival in Patients with Intracranial Tumors: Neuronavigation, MRI, and 5-ALA

Luis Fernando Moura da Silva,
Guilherme Augusto de Souza Machado and Ricardo Ramina

Abstract

This chapter describes the usefulness of surgical technologies such as intraoperative MRI, 5-ALA fluorescence-guided surgery, and neuronavigation as tools to make brain tumor resections safer and more effective. The focuses are practical aspects and the relevant literature regarding the impact of their use in avoidance of complications, improvement in survival rates, and some tips and tricks acquired in the experience of our department. All three strategies have an important role in neuro-oncological surgery. The future probably will prove that the combination of these tools, selected case by case, is the best way to achieve the best results regarding safety and effectiveness.

Keywords: neurosurgical procedures, brain neoplasms, neuronavigation, fluorescence-guided surgery, magnetic resonance imaging

1. Introduction

In all areas of science and knowledge, technology development is thought to bring solutions that optimize process, reduce costs, and make things safer. Brain tumor resection is a routine procedure in neurosurgical practice. In most of the cases, complete surgical resection remains as the gold standard of treatment. But some cases are real challenges to the neurosurgical team. Deep-seated tumors demand planned pathways to achieve it considering functions of each area of the brain, including white fiber tracts to avoid injury related to the approach. Besides eloquent area involvement, in some cases, despite simple or complex approaches, some aspects of the lesion turns them more difficult to resect such as its consistency, adherence to neighboring structures, and the presence of a well-defined cleavage plan. Neurosurgery has this cardinal aspect that every structure matters and injuries can bring catastrophic consequences.

Depending on the aggressiveness of the tumor, the tolerance to incomplete resection changes. But, for example, in benign tumors with incomplete resection, remnants can be followed by the "watch-and-wait" policy. Only in case of progression, a new decision should be done: reoperation, complementary treatment such

IntechOpen

as radiosurgery, radiotherapy, chemotherapy, or immunotherapy (depending on its characteristics). In cases of malignant tumors such as gliomas and metastasis, the extent of resection (EOR) is directly related to recurrence and survival. Incomplete resection for these patients should be only discussed if the risk of neurological injury is high. Obviously, *not to harm* is always the most important principle. Increase in survival only makes sense if accompanied by quality.

Even with intense microsurgical training, the multidisciplinary treatment challenge remains. Some strategies such as intraoperative monitoring, awake surgery, and intraoperative histology (margin biopsy) can be used to improve the goal. In this chapter neuronavigation, intraoperative magnet resonance imaging (ioMRI), and 5-aminolevulinic acid (5-ALA) are discussed as tools to improve the safety and efficacy of intracranial tumor resection.

2. Neuronavigation

Neuronavigation has a fundamental role in contemporary neurosurgery. This tool allowed surgeons to better individualize treatment tailoring craniotomies and localizing structures or lesions intraoperatively. It consists of a frameless stereotactic system of localization based on pre- or intraoperative image data. The data used can be a fusion of different techniques like CT, MRI anatomical or functional sequences, US, or PET-CT.

The most important indications of the use of navigation are planning of craniotomy, intraoperative localization of lesions or structures, and guided biopsies.

2.1 Craniotomy planning

Using metastasis as an example, neurosurgeons increasingly attempt to resect as much tumor tissue as possible to impact disease control and survival. If a patient has four metastases of 4 centimeters that can be completely resected, this procedure should be indicated. Even if multiple craniotomies are needed, this should not dissuade the surgeon to indicate it [1]. In these special cases, considering that these metastases are in different places of the brain, neuronavigation makes a real difference with a tailored and focused approach to each lesion.

Neuronavigation allows direct access to the lesions, even if small, reducing the size of craniotomy, dural opening, unwanted manipulation of the brain, duration of surgery, blood loss, volume of the tissue to be healed, length of stay in the hospital, recurrence rate, time to be available for complementary treatment if needed, and costs and improving recurrence-free survival (RFS) and performance status [2, 3].

In cases of ventricular endoscopic approach, neuronavigation can also be very useful. Some patients with pineal or third ventricle-located tumors with noncommunicating hydrocephalus, for example, need third ventriculostomy and biopsy. In order to offer a direct straightforward approach, avoiding lesions of related structures, two different trepanations/small craniotomies can be performed guided by neuronavigation (**Figure 1**).

Besides defining the position of the craniotomy, still regarding surgical approach, neuronavigation can help in many ways to improve safety of neurosurgical procedures. Identification of sinus position in retrosigmoid craniotomy has been demonstrated successfully avoiding unnecessary sinus exposition reducing complications [4]. Also, superficial vein identification before dural opening was demonstrated, eliminating the need to use indocyanine to make a transdural analysis, for

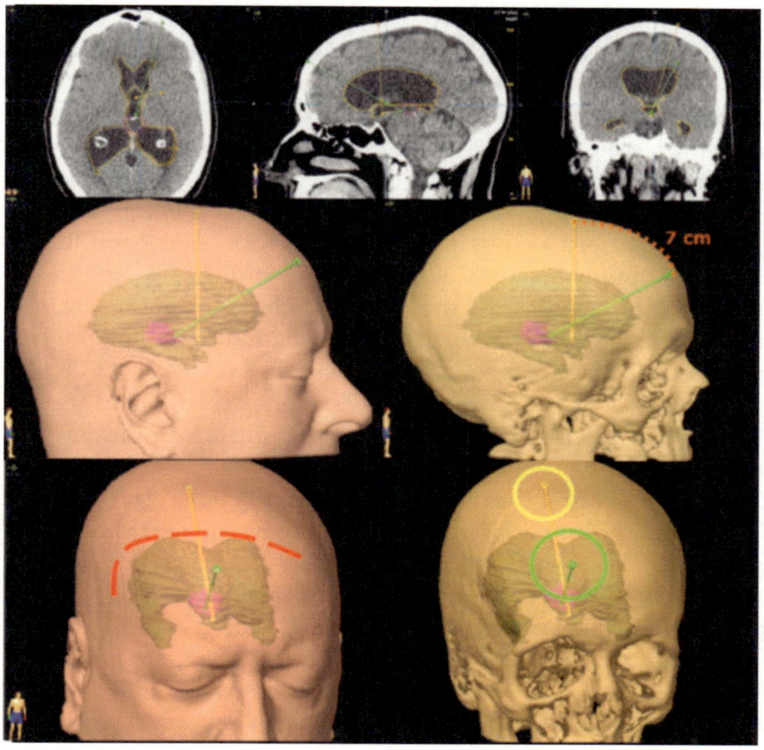

Figure 1.
Patient with indication of a third ventricle lesion and third ventriculostomy. Neuronavigation plan of two different craniotomies to straightforward approach avoiding critical structures. The yellow trajectory with direct approach to Monro's foramen and Liliequist membrane. The green target to direct approach of a third ventricle lesion. Approaches point distant 7 cm. Two small craniotomies were preferred and successfully achieved their targets.

example [5]. These strategies reduce also the risk of bleeding and venous closure, which can have a negative impact on surgical outcome.

2.2 Intraoperative localization of structures/lesions

When used to localize superficial lesions/anatomical structures and tailor surgical approach, neuronavigation has high accuracy, being a very reliable tool, because the intracranial compartment remains untouched. However, the main drawback of neuronavigation is that it is not a real-time evaluation.

The accuracy between preoperative images and real intraoperative anatomy is influenced during many surgical steps that result in dislocation of structures, called brain shift. Several surgical aspects are not related to wrong landmark selection, hardware movement, or software algorithm influence on brain shift. The causes are classified as physical (hardware movement, patient position, and gravity), surgical (fluid loss, tissue loss, and surgical equipment), and biological (mannitol and tumor type) [6].

The effect of gravity is an important physical factor of brain shift. It interacts with two surgical causes: fluid loss and tissue loss. After tumor resection or relevant CSF drainage, adjacent healthy tissue becomes unsupported with sagging of the brain. Loss of 20 cm^3 of CSF in deep brain stimulation (DBS) surgery was demonstrated to result in the shift of the anterior commissure by approximately 2 mm [7]. Mannitol administration during surgery also can influence, especially in cases where high intracranial pressure levels or large edema are present. Neuronavigation does not contraindicate the administration of mannitol. But its use should be used judiciously, not routinely. Regarding biological causes, some authors observed an association between tumor biology and unique patterns of the shift. But the reasons are not well understood, and more studies should analyze this before generalization can be made [6].

Previously, many attempts to identify intra-axial tumor margins using neuronavigation were performed, but it could be done with reliable results due to brain shift. Other options such as fluorescence and ioMRI have superior results. Otherwise, targets located in fixed structures like the bone, brainstem, and skull base meninges tolerate better intracranial manipulation. The dural implantation of a skull base meningioma, for example, can be checked with navigation during the procedure, because it will suffer few the effect of brain shift. But as accuracy should be low, the shift needs to be weighted in every procedure. In brainstem biopsies, the passage of the biopsy needle through the parenchyma does not change target position significantly; but if the trajectory accidentally passes through the ventricle with CSF drainage, the brain shift can have significant influence hindering correct target achievement.

Correction of brain shift can be done using intraoperative MRI to update the navigation; or other real-time exams, where ioMRI is not available, can be performed to compare and adjust it such as ultrasound (US) [2, 8].

Ultrasound is a fast, cheap, real-time, and commonly available exam. Although its image quality is not comparable to MRI, it plays an important role in brain tumor surgery. After craniotomy, for example, brain shift can occur even if brain deformation is still not present. Placing the probe directly on the dura and superimposing identifiable structures on both techniques can confirm if neuronavigation is still adequate. The main concept of using intraoperative US is that the focus is not on diagnosis but on localization. Undoubtedly, MRI is the gold standard exam to analyze brain lesions and define diagnosis. But to locate lesions and some structures, US is sometimes enough with the advantage of being easily and real-time performed. ioUS can affect the decision of further resection in 59% of cases [9]. Association of these two techniques offers the possibility to overcome the limitations of each one separately improving the safety of the procedure (**Figure 2**).

Another important intraoperative use of navigation is in the association with other tools such as awake surgery and transcranial magnetic stimulation (TMS). Navigated TMS-based DTI-fiber tracking in awake surgery has been demonstrated

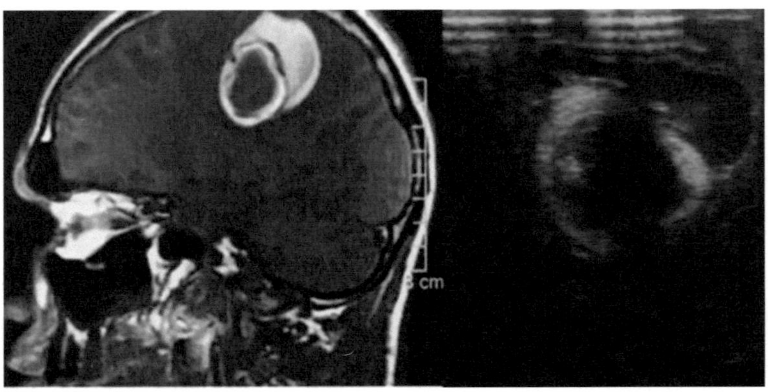

Figure 2.
MRI of a hemorrhagic tumor with ioUS view. Easy identification of both limits and differences of cystic and solid components.

as a useful tool in the treatment of highly eloquent gliomas with results considering craniotomy size, EOR, duration of surgery, postoperative deficits, Karnofsky Performance Scale (KPS), and length of stay in the hospital [10]. Association of image-guided resection of glioblastoma in eloquent brain areas facilitated by laser surface thermal therapy was also demonstrated with favorable long-term results. This strategy allowed the higher rates of complete resection and improved overall survival without the negative effect on postoperative functional status [11].

2.3 Guided biopsy

Biopsy of intracranial lesion is an important diagnostic tool in neurosurgery. With the progression of genetic and molecular characterization of tumors, biopsy becomes even more important in deep-seated lesions with difficult access such as in the thalamus, brainstem, and pineal gland.

Frame-based intracranial biopsy has been the gold standard technique for intracranial biopsy for a long time. The stereotactic system provides excellent precision of target achievement. After development of neuronavigation, the frameless intracranial biopsy, guided by neurosurgery, has evolved a lot. Both methods have similar effectiveness to histological diagnosis. But a frameless system has become increasingly the first choice among neurosurgeons due to reduced equipment size; reduced work of calculations to define targets, entry point, and trajectory; patient's comfort; reduced surgical time with navigation; and the absence of the need to redo image examination after placement of the frame (**Figure 3**) [12].

The use of real-time ioMRI-guided biopsy has also been compared to frame-based and frameless neuronavigation-guided biopsy with comparable diagnostic yield in patients with no prior treatment. ioMRI-guided biopsy was associated with short hospital stay [12]. But ioMRI is not available in many places, and navigation-guided frameless biopsy continues as the first option in most departments.

In pineal tumors, as some patients have hydrocephalus, endoscopic biopsy associated with third ventriculostomy is a feasible option, as cited before.

The most common complications of deep biopsies are brain shift, hemorrhage, and failure in representativeness of samples. Brain shift was discussed before in Section 2.2. Hemorrhage can be directly related to biopsy (intratumoral) or to the trajectory

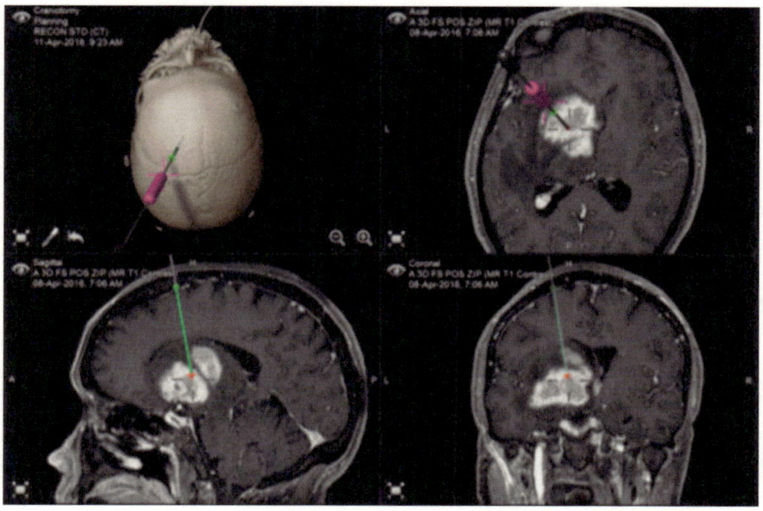

Figure 3.
MRI of a frameless-based biopsy (neuronavigation guided) of a deep-seated lesion. Trajectory planning without any passage through ventricular system to avoid CSF drainage and brain shift.

(needle track). Hemorrhage is avoided with preoperative evaluation of coagulation marking a trajectory that avoids any arterial or venous structure that is achieved by using multiplanar reconstruction of image [13]. Representativeness of sample has been traditionally analyzed with adequate target definition in image and intraoperative pathology/frozen section. More recently fluorescence has been associated with biopsy procedures with good correlation compared to frozen section to check acquisition of relevant samples. Both 5-ALA and fluorescein were evaluated [14, 15].

3. Magnet resonance imaging (MRI)

In neuro-oncological surgery, complete resection with preservation of functions and quality of life is normally the goal of the procedure. Defining complete resection intraoperatively is easier in extra-axial tumors than in intra-axial tumors such as low-grade gliomas. A surgeon's perception of gross total resection (GTR) usually relies on the visual and tactile aspects of tumor boundaries. Studies compared the surgeon's perception with imaging findings and determined inaccuracy and overestimation of intraoperative EOR by up to a factor of 3 [16–18]. Young adult patients with low-grade glioma who undergo a neurosurgeon-determined GTR have a higher than 50% risk of tumor progression in 5 years postoperatively [18].

The surgeon's experience also was not significant to define additional resection. The positive predictive value (PPV) of the surgeon's expectation was shown to be high (93.1%). On the other hand, and most importantly, the ability to exclude additional resection from the intraoperative impression was very low (43.6%) [19].

This is a major concern specially in tumors that EOR is proven to be related with recurrence and survival.

Intraoperative or transoperative MRI emerges exactly in this context to clearly determine if GTR was achieved or not. Literature suggests rates of further operative resection secondary to ioMRI evaluation range from 13.3 to 59.37%, confirming the impact of this tool on the extent of tumor resection [20, 21].

Analysis comparing EOR, GTR, and progression-free survival (PFS) and overall survival (OS) in patients with gliomas that underwent ioMRI also confirmed the benefit with improvement of these aspects. The author showed an increase in GTR rate of 24.1%. In 59.37% of cases that underwent ioMRI, further resection was needed [21]. Certainty of ioMRI can make surgeon more tolerant and relaxed, ending resection early relying on ioMRI evaluation. But even if this is considered, the improve in resection is substantial.

In complex located tumors, for example, insular gliomas, ioMRI check during awake craniotomy increased EOR in 15.1%. Considering that median EOR on ioMRI was 51.2% and after further resection was 84.5%, it is clear that ioMRI really impacts outcome [22].

Identification of margins is not always simple. It depends on the tumor type, MRI sequence analyzed, and surgical trauma with blood-brain barrier break. In cases of high-grade glioma surgery, PWI helps in identification of tumoral x non-tumoral tissue. Another option is the use of a single layer of oxidized regenerated cellulose covering the cavity to enhance margin visualization in ioMRI. Being a hemostatic agent, it accelerates oxidation of oxyhemoglobin to metahemoglobin, which is paramagnetic, and, so, it has a hyperintense signal in T1 sequences. This layer of hyperintense line observed may be a useful marker of tumor resection borders in cerebral glioma surgery [23].

Pituitary tumors also benefit from ioMRI. A systematic review observed that complete radiological resection in patients whose procedure involved intraoperative ultrasound was 67.1% (range 63.5–77.8%) and endocrine remission was 88.4% (range

76–100%) [24]. Studies with ioMRI also evidences the benefits with intraoperative unexpected residuals in up to 42% (range 15–83%) of cases, of which re-exploration was attempted in 36% (range 9–83%) and further tumor resection occurred in 33% (range 9–83%) of the cases [25]. But this paper considered low- and high-field ioMRI. In a study with 3 T ioMR, a complete resection was observed in 69% of the cases.

Intraoperative image interpretation is even more difficult in transsphenoidal pituitary surgery than in glioma surgery, for example. This evaluation should only be done by an experienced neuroradiologist, because the literature shows relevant cases of false-positive leading to resection of normal tissue, in both ioMRI and ioUS [24, 25]. The Congress of Neurological Surgeons (CNS) suggested in 2016 that intraoperative images in nonfunctioning adenomas may help to improve overall gross total resection but at the cost of removing normal tissue [26]. So, we suggest weighting cost-benefit relation differently in nonfunctioning x functioning adenomas. But in an experienced team, good results can be achieved.

In the beginning, ioMRI started with low-field strengths of 0.2–0.5 T. These units, although cheaper and requiring less spaces, take longer to perform scanning and produce low-quality images when compared to high-field (1.5 T and higher) equipment. Besides this, the possibility of advanced images such as DTI favors the use of high-field equipment [27, 28].

Cost is one of the most limiting factors to the spread of ioMRI. Additionally, the price of the whole equipment and software and surgical and anesthesia equipment should be developed to be compatible with ioMRI environment. These adapted equipment are also expensive, which increases even more the investment on a magnet dedicated exclusively to intraoperative images. Besides this, in few years MRI equipment becomes obsolete with the need to change to maintain it updated.

In order to overcome this limitation, the concept of "outside MRI" was proposed by Ramina et al. in 2010. In this strategy after completing the resection, oxidized regenerated cellulose is put to cover surgical cavity, and a partial closure of the dura is performed. The exposed dura is covered with cottonoid plates, and the skin is closed with running suture. A sterile plastic sheet covers the entire head to assure sterility and complete the preparation for MRI. The patient is conducted in the MRI-compatible bed through an internal special lift, designed for this purpose, to the MRI facilities. Time required to whole exam, since patient left OR and came back, was 25 min. No infection was observed [29]. Ahmadi et al. recently confirmed that inside ioMRI did not increase complications (hemorrhage, wound healing, and infection) in glioma surgery. In their publication the ioMRI procedure time was higher with a mean of 57 min [30]. "Outside MRI" has all advantages of "inside models" and the additional advantage of integrating neurosurgery/neuroradiology teams, which may lead to better results [29].

4. 5-Aminolevulinic acid

5-ALA is a prodrug and leads to accumulation of protoporphyrin IX (PPIX) in gliomas and other tumor cells by an interaction with heme biosynthesis process. With special filters and blue/violet light, it is possible to see fluorescence of PPIX as light red or an intense pinkish color in a dark blue background. These filters and lights are usually part or an upgrade of surgical microscope. Normal brain tissue does not induce PPIX expression after ALA administration, and a high selectivity of malignant glioma cells is observed. When density of tumor cells in the tissue is above 10%, fluorescence is expected to be present [31].

This is another tool to go further with the concept that tumor tissues are many times much more than what we see with normal light surgical microscopy or even contrast-enhanced MRI. A high association between contrast enhancement and PPIX fluorescence is observed. But it was shown that PPIX fluorescence in non-contrast-enhanced areas can be present with good correlation with the presence of tumor tissue. So, PPIX accumulations seem to be more sensitive to glioma detection than contrast-agent accumulation (**Figure 4**) [31, 32].

Fluoroethyl tyrosine PET has been demonstrated to have a good correlation with PPIX fluorescence in gliomas without typical glioblastoma imaging features [33]. Also, areas with high atypia in low grade or non-contrast enhancing in high grade suggested by PET could be confirmed with 5-ALA fluorescence. The explanation to these findings may be in the mechanism of each method. Contrast enhancement and sodium-fluorescein fluorescence have intraoperative correlation, and both occur due to disruption of blood-brain barrier, which is not specific from tumors. 5-ALA fluorescence and PET tracer uptake, in turn, occur due to specific metabolism of tumor tissue. 5-ALA may be even more special than PET because it does not consider only the general quantitative aspect of metabolism and goes beyond. Its mechanism relates to a metabolic phenomenon of a pathway typical from a tumor tissue and not from a normal tissue [34].

Other tumors than WHO IV gliomas have also been tested regarding fluorescence after 5-ALA administration. Literature shows results with approximately 15–20% of fluorescence with 5-ALA in low-grade gliomas, 85–100% in high-grade gliomas, and 55–80% in metastasis [32, 35, 36]. In our most recent data analysis from INC, we could observe 5-ALA-positive fluorescence in 97.7% cases of WHO IV gliomas, 90% cases of WHO III gliomas, 22.2% cases of WHO II gliomas, and 85.7% in cases of metastasis. The quality of fluorescence differs among tumor types. In low-grade gliomas, for example, with positive fluorescence we observed usually weak to mild with stronger foci in some cases (higher atypia); metastasis, on the other hand, usually shows mild to strong fluorescence (**Figure 5**).

During the procedure, the surgeon alternates between white light resection and blue/violet light resection. This is important because white light shows anatomy, structures, and blood better. Only the resection, specially boundaries, is guided by fluorescence. Blood, inclusive, may be a confounding factor, because it prevents the

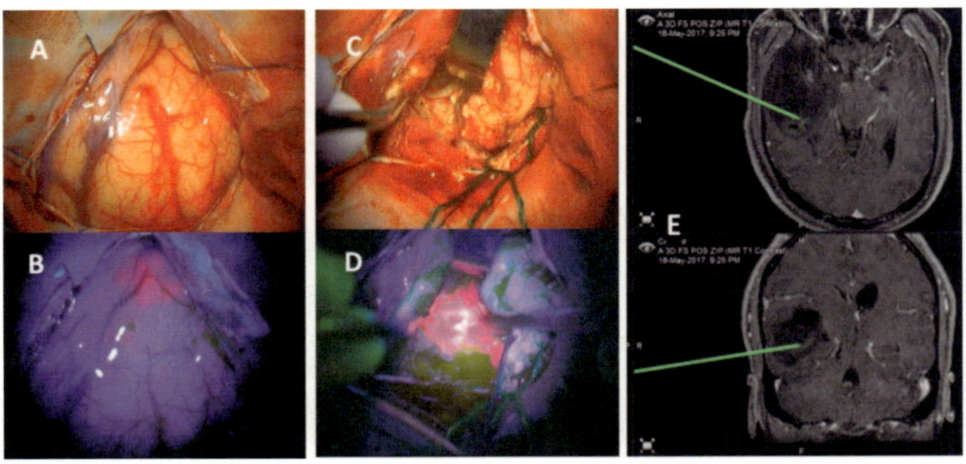

Figure 4.
Glioma patient operated on using 5-ALA. A and B show white light and blue-filter images with identifiable tumoral tissue on the cortex, clearly visible with blue filter and difficult to identify with white light. C and D show areas of tumor with intense fluorescence in blue filter, corresponding to contrast-enhanced area shown by neuronavigation in E.

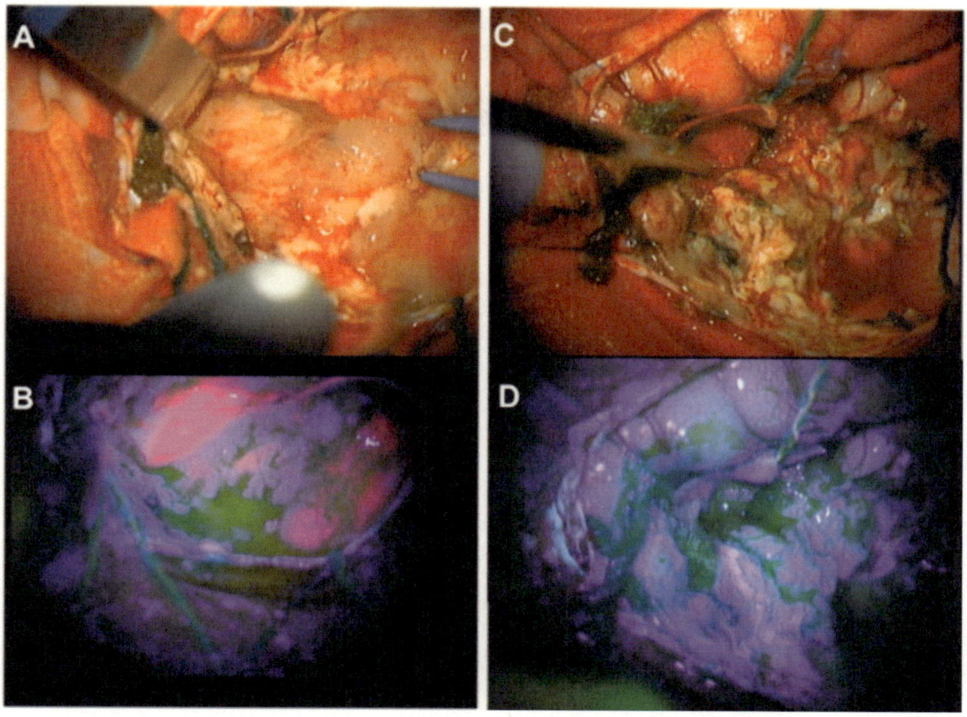

Figure 5.
High-grade glioma patient operated on using 5-ALA. A and B show white light and blue-filter images with clearly identifiable tumoral tissue. In blue-filter image, a reddish color is observed, confirming the presence of tumoral tissue. The pinkish image demonstrates areas with tumoral infiltration. C and D show complete resection without any identifiable tumor in both white light and blue-filter images. Normal tissue appears blueish.

visualization of fluorescence. So, an adequate size of craniotomy (allowing light to enter the deep surgical field) and hemostasis (to avoid a blood layer over tumor area) in 5-ALA-guided surgery are more than ever must-do concepts. More common collateral effects are transient increase in liver enzymes and light sensitivity of the skin until 24 h after administration.

A combination of techniques may be the future of fluorescence-guided surgery. Dual-labeling surgery using 5-ALA and fluorescein has been tested with interesting results. Fluorescein created a useful background for 5-ALA fluorescence. It appeared as orange to red surrounded by greenly fluorescent normal brain and edematous tissue. Unspecific extravasation of fluorescein at resection margins was also observed, which did not interfere with 5-ALA fluorescence detection [37].

EOR and 6-month PFS have been proven to increase with the use of 5-ALA in cases of malignant gliomas. PFS at 6 months was 41% in 5-ALA group x 21.1% in the group operated only with white light-based resection. EOR improved from 36% in white light-based resection to 65% in 5-ALA [38]. EOR has also been analyzed in a systematic review with 22 series from the literature, including 1163 patients, with a GTR rate of 66.2% in gliomas using 5-ALA [35].

Other non-fluorescence techniques can also help in combination with 5-ALA. Intraoperative cortical stimulation added new advantages to resection about the function of tissues and provided additional safety for resection of primary malignant tumor in eloquent areas [39]. Intraoperative 3D US, as well as ioMRI, also was demonstrated to bring different information that when combined with 5-ALA fluorescence can improve the extent of resection, especially in non-enhancing tumors [9, 31, 40].

A comparison of combined ioMRI + 5-ALA versus ioMRI isolated in patients with high grade (WHO IV) gliomas showed that in combined group EOR above 95% was reached in all cases. In the ioMRI group, 18% of EOR were below 95% with a minimum EOR of 87% in this group versus a minimum EOR of 97% in the combined group [40]. Considering that EOR of 78% is the cutoff to improve survival in high-grade gliomas, both methods were efficient. But the association of 5-ALA and ioMRI leads to a higher rate, possibly having a greater impact on survival. But this is still to be proven, demanding further studies.

Despite drawbacks of being only a 2D information, hidden 5-ALA fluorescence by blood or hemostatic agents, and regulatory issues in many countries, 5-ALA-guided resection is a very useful tool offering real-time information from the tissue (not indirectly not from images), without the influence of brain shift avoiding second-look procedures or even new complementary resections, which are usually much more expensive than the costs of 5-ALA (**Figure 5**).

5. Conclusion

Every tool that can add data to surgical planning or intraoperative evaluation is valid. Neuronavigation is very useful in surgical strategy (planning and intraoperative steps) improving efficacy and safety of the procedure. 5-ALA-guided resection and intraoperative image (such as ioUS and ioMRI) are proven to be cost-effective with increased GTR rates and an impact on survival. The future probably will prove that combination of these tools, selected case by case, is the best way to achieve the best results regarding safety and effectiveness.

Conflict of interest

Authors have no conflict of interest.

Author details

Luis Fernando Moura da Silva[1,2]*, Guilherme Augusto de Souza Machado[1] and Ricardo Ramina[1]

1 Neurological Institute of Curitiba—INC, Curitiba, Brazil

2 NOZ Neurocentro, São Luis, Brazil

*Address all correspondence to: luisfernando@inc-neuro.com.br

IntechOpen

© 2019 The Author(s). Licensee IntechOpen. This chapter is distributed under the terms of the Creative Commons Attribution License (http://creativecommons.org/licenses/by/3.0), which permits unrestricted use, distribution, and reproduction in any medium, provided the original work is properly cited. (cc) BY

References

[1] Lee JJ. Surgical treatment of multiple brain metastases. Journal of Neurosurgery. 1993;**79**:210-216

[2] Hu S, Kang H, Baek Y, El FG, Kuang A, Choi HS. Real-time imaging of brain tumor for image-guided surgery. Advanced Healthcare Materials. Aug 2018;7(16):e1800066

[3] Bir SC, Konar SK, Maiti TK, Thakur JD, Guthikonda B, Nanda A. Utility of neuronavigation in intracranial meningioma resection: A single-center retrospective study. World Neurosurgery. 2016;**90**:546-555

[4] da Silva EB, Leal AG, Milano JB, da Silva LFM, Clemente RS, Ramina R. Image-guided surgical planning using anatomical landmarks in the retrosigmoid approach. Acta Neurochirurgica. 2010;**152**(5):905-910

[5] Ricciardi L, Maria G, Pepa D, Izzo A, Simboli GA, Polli FM, et al. Use of neuronavigation system for superficial vein identification: Safe and quick method to avoid intraoperative bleeding and vein closure: Technical note. World Neurosurgery. 2018;**117**:92-96

[6] Gerard IJ, Kersten-oertel M, Petrecca K, Sirhan D, Hall JA, Collins DL. Brain shift in neuronavigation of brain tumors: A review. Medical Image Analysis. 2017;**35**:403-420

[7] Elias WJ, Fu K-M, Frysinger RC. Cortical and subcortical brain shift during stereotactic procedures. Journal of Neurosurgery. 2007;**107**:983-988

[8] Prada F, Del Bene M, Mattei L, Lodigiani L, DeBeni S, Kolev V, et al. Preoperative magnetic resonance and intraoperative ultrasound fusion imaging for real-time neuronavigation in brain tumor surgery—Präoperative MRI-und intraoperative Ultraschallfusion für die Echtzeit-Neuronavigation in der Neurochirurgie von Hirntumoren. Ultraschall in der Medizin. 2015;**36**:174-186

[9] Moiyadi AV, Shetty PM. Usefulness of three-dimensional navigable intraoperative ultrasound in resection of brain tumors with a special emphasis on malignant gliomas. Acta Neurochirurgica. 2013;**155**:2217-2225

[10] Sollmann N, Kelm A, Ille S, Schröder A, Zimmer C, Ringel F, et al. Setup presentation and clinical outcome analysis of treating highly language-eloquent gliomas via preoperative navigated transcranial magnetic stimulation and tractography. Neurosurgical Focus. 2018;**44**(6):E2

[11] Rozumenko A, Kliuchka V, Rozumenko V, Semenova V, Kolesnyk S, Fedorenko Z. Image-guided resection of glioblastoma in eloquent brain areas facilitated by laser surface thermal therapy: Clinical outcomes and long-term results. Neurosurgical Review. 2018;**41**(4):1045-1052

[12] Lu Y, Yeung C, Radmanesh A, Wiemann R, Black PM, Golby AJ, et al. Comparative effectiveness of frame-based, frameless and intraoperative MRI guided brain biopsy techniques. World Neurosurgery. 2015;**83**(3):261-268

[13] Abdel A, Shakal S, Abdel E, Mokbel H. Hemorrhage after stereotactic biopsy from intra-axial brain lesions: Incidence and avoidance. Journal of Neurological Surgery Part A: Central European Neurosurgery. 2014;**75**:177-182

[14] Kiesel B, Millesi M, Woehrer A, Furtner J, Bavand A, Roetzer T, et al. 5-ALA-induced fluorescence as a marker for diagnostic tissue in stereotactic biopsies of intracranial lymphomas: Experience in 41 patients. Neurosurgical Focus. 2018;**44**(6):E7

[15] Thien A, Han JX, Kumar K, Ng YP, Rao JP, Ng WH. Investigation of the usefulness of fluorescein sodium fluorescence in stereotactic brain biopsy. Acta Neurochirurgica. 2018;**160**(2):317-324

[16] Renfrow JJ, Strowd RE, Laxton AW, Tatter SB, Geer CP, Lesser GJ. Surgical considerations in the optimal management of patients with malignant brain tumors. Current Treatment Options in Oncology. 2017;**18**(8):46

[17] Orringer D, Lau D, Khatri S, Zamora-Berridi GJ, Zhang K, Wu C, et al. Extent of resection in patients with glioblastoma: Limiting factors, perception of resectability, and effect on survival. Journal of Neurosurgery. 2012;**117**:851-859

[18] Shaw EG, Berkey B, Coons SW, Bullerd D, Brachman D, Buckner JC, et al. Recurrence following neurosurgeon-determined gross-total resection of adult supratentorial low-grade glioma: Results of a prospective clinical trial. Journal of Neurosurgery. 2008;**109**:835-841

[19] Scherer M, Jungk C, Younsi A, Kickingereder P, Müller S, Unterberg A. Factors triggering an additional resection and determining residual tumor volume on intraoperative MRI: Analysis from a prospective single-center registry of supratentorial gliomas. Neurosurgical Focus. 2016;**40**(3):E4

[20] Swinney C, Li A, Bhatti I, Veeravagu A. Optimization of tumor resection with intra-operative magnetic resonance imaging. Journal of Clinical Neuroscience. 2016;**34**:11-14

[21] Familiari P, Frati A, Pesce A, Miscusi M, Cimatti M, Raco A. Real impact of intraoperative MRI in newly diagnosed glioblastoma multiforme resection: An observational analytic cohort study from a single surgeon experience. World Neurosurgery. 2018;**116**:e9-e17

[22] Motomura K, Natsume A, Iijima K, Kuramitsu S, Fujii M, Yamamoto T, et al. Surgical benefits of combined awake craniotomy and intraoperative magnetic resonance imaging for gliomas associated with eloquent areas. Journal of Neurosurgery. 2017;**127**:790-797

[23] Ramina R, Coelho Neto M, Nascimento AB, Vosgerau R. Intraoperative MRI features of absorbable oxidized regenerated cellulose during cerebral glioma surgery. Brazilian Neurosurgery. 2013;**24**(1):16-10

[24] Marcus HJ, Vercauteren T, Ourselin S, Dorward NL. Literature review intraoperative ultrasound in patients undergoing transsphenoidal surgery for pituitary adenoma: Systematic review. World Neurosurgery. 2017;**106**:680-685

[25] Chittiboina P. iMRI during transsphenoidal surgery. Neurosurgery Clinics of North America. 2017;**28**(4):499-512

[26] Aghi MK, Chen CC, Fleseriu M, Lucas JW, Kuo JS, Barkhoudarian G, et al. Congress of neurological surgeons systematic review and evidence-based guidelines on the management of patients with nonfunctioning pituitary adenomas: Executive summary. Neurosurgery. 2016;**79**(4):521-523

[27] Bisdas S, Roder C, Ernemann U, Tatagiba MS. Intraoperative MR imaging in neurosurgery. Clinical Neuroradiology. 2015;**25**:237-244

[28] Rao G. Intraoperative MRI and maximizing extent of resection. Neurosurgery Clinics of North America. 2017;**28**(4):477-485

[29] Ramina R, Neto MC, Giacomelli A, Barros E Jr, Vosgerau R, Nascimento A, et al. Optimizing costs of intraoperative

magnetic resonance imaging. A series of 29 glioma cases. Acta Neurochirurgica. 2010;**152**:27-33

[30] Ahmadi R, Campos B, Haux D, Rieke J, Beigel B, Unterberg A. Assessing perioperative complications associated with use of intraoperative magnetic resonance imaging during glioma surgery—A single centre experience with 516 cases. British Journal of Neurosurgery. 2016;**30**(4):397-400

[31] Molina ES, Schipmann S, Stummer W. Maximizing safe resections: The roles of 5-aminolevulinic acid and intraoperative MR imaging in glioma surgery—Review of the literature. Neurosurgical Review. 2017 [Epub ahead of print]

[32] Stummer W, Suero Molina E. Fluorescence imaging/agents in tumor resection. Neurosurgery Clinics of North America. 2017;**28**(4):569-583

[33] Jaber M, Wölfer J, Ewelt C, Holling M, Hasselblatt M, Niederstadt T, et al. 5-Aminolevulinic acid in low-grade gliomas and high-grade gliomas lacking glioblastoma imaging features: An analysis based on fluorescence, magnetic resonance imaging, 18F-fluoroethyl tyrosine positron emission tomography, and tumor molecular factors. Neurosurgery. 2016;**78**(3):401-411

[34] Yano H, Nakayama N, Ohe N, Miwa K, Shinoda J, Iwama T. Pathological analysis of the surgical margins of resected glioblastomas excised using photodynamic visualization with both 5-aminolevulinic acid and fluorescein sodium. Journal of Neuro-Oncology. 2017;**133**:389-397

[35] Ferraro N, Barbarite E, Albert TR, Berchmans E, Shah AH, Bregy A, et al. The role of 5-aminolevulinic acid in brain tumor surgery: A systematic review. Neurosurgical Review. 2016;**39**(4):545-555

[36] Ramina R, da Silva EB Jr, Coelho Neto M, Ruschel LG, Navarrette FAC. 5-aminolevulinic acid—Protoporphyrin IX fluorescence-guided surgery for CNS tumors. First 41 cases in Latin America. Brazilian Neurosurgery. 2017;**27**(1):13-19

[37] Molina ES, Wölfer J, Ewelt C, Ehrhardt A, Brokinkel B, Stummer W. Dual-labeling with 5-aminolevulinic acid and fluorescein for fluorescence-guided resection of high-grade gliomas: Technical note. Journal of Neurosurgery. 2018;**128**:399-405

[38] Stummer W, Pichlmeier U, Meinel T, Wiestler OD, Zanella F, Reulen H. Fluorescence-guided surgery with 5-aminolevulinic acid for resection of malignant glioma: A randomised controlled multicentre phase III trial. The Lancet Oncology. 2006;**7**:392-401

[39] Feigl GC, Ritz R, Moraes M, Klein J, Ramina K, Gharabaghi A, et al. Resection of malignant brain tumors in eloquent cortical areas: A new multimodal approach combining 5-aminolevulinic acid and intraoperative monitoring. Journal of Neurosurgery. 2010;**113**:352-357

[40] Coburger J, Hagel V, Wirtz CR, König R. Surgery for glioblastoma: Impact of the combined use of 5-aminolevulinic acid and intraoperative MRI on extent of resection and survival. PLoS One. 2015;**10**(2):e0131872

Section 3

Management of Specific Tumors

Chapter 5

Management of Refractory/Aggressive Pituitary Adenomas Review of Current Treatment Options

Congxin Dai, Xiaohai Liu, Sihai Ma, Ming Feng, Xinjie Bao, Kan Deng, Yong Yao, Renzhi Wang, DX. Feng, E. Fonkem, Frank Y. Shan and Jason H. Huang

Abstract

Tumors of central nervous system (CNS) account for a small portion of tumors of human body, which includes tumors occurring in the parenchyma of brain and spinal cord as well as their coverings. This chapter covers some new development in some major brain tumors in both pediatric and adult populations, as well as some uncommon but diagnostic and management challenging tumors.

Keywords: refractory pituitary adenoma, macroadenoma and microadenoma, trans-sphenoidal adenomectomy, targeting therapy

1. Introduction

The anterior pituitary gland (adenohypophysis) is an important organ for human development and physiological functions (so called "Master Gland"), which comprises several different cell types, responsible for the synthesis and secretion of a specific hormone or group of specific hormones (plurihormonal), such as growth hormone (GH), adrenocorticotrophic hormone (ACTH), and prolactin (PRL). Each of these cell types may give rise to a discrete pituitary adenoma (PA) subtype that is either hormonal active (functional) or inactive (nonfunctional).

As one of the most common pituitary neuroendocrine tumors, pituitary adenomas (PAs) constitute the overwhelming majority of tumors arising in the pituitary gland and account for 10–15% intracranial neoplasms. Incidental microadenoma (smaller than 10 mm in diameter) may occur in up to 27% of pituitary glands examined at autopsy, and up to one-fifth of the human population has pituitary abnormalities on magnetic resonance imaging (MRI).

Majority of PAs are benign and slow growing; however, up to 10% of PAs are aggressive with invasive growth and can exhibit clinical abnormal behavior with high rates of recurrences [1]. Based on the recent WHO classification in 2017, a more detailed tumor classification by immunohistochemical stain (IHC) was proposed, which identifies a subset of PAs with aggressive clinical behavior characterized by clinical recurrence, which includes PAs with elevated Ki-67 proliferation

IntechOpen

index, sparsely granulated somatotroph PAs, Lactotroph PAs in men, silent corticotroph PAs, Crooke cell PAs, and plurihormonal PAs with PIT-1 positivity. PIT-1 is one of the pituitary transcription factors, sometimes to be used to clarify the PAs' tumor linages.

Clinically, a subset of aggressive PAs characterized with high Ki-67 index, rapid growth, frequent recurrence, and resistant to conventional treatments is defined as refractory PAs [2]. These refractory PAs often have a very poor prognosis and even with an occasionally fatal outcome; however, there is no general agreement about how to manage the patient with refractory PAs. For neurosurgeons and clinicians, it is difficult to optimally choose the therapeutic options in treatment of refractory PAs in order to improve the prognoses of these patients; it is very important and necessary to review the emerging treatments for refractory PAs. This chapter is going to review some current treatment options for those refractory PAs.

2. Management of refractory PAs by surgical treatment

Typically, multimodal approaches are required for managing refractory PAs. Except prolactin-secreting adenomas (prolactinomas), which should be first treated with dopamine agonists (DAs), the primary treatment option is usually surgery, even surgery is usually unable to cure or control the refractory PAs [3]. However, the therapeutic goals of surgery are maximum reduction of tumor mass, decompression of visual pathways, best possible reduction of hormonal oversecretion, amelioration of clinical symptoms, and minimization of complications [4].

Most of the refractory PAs are largely invasive, infiltrating adjacent tissues; repeated surgery seldom achieves complete tumor excision. However, surgical resection is still necessary to relieve compressive symptoms [5].

Repeated trans-sphenoidal surgery is generally more difficult to perform than the initial operation due to the increased risk of morbidity and mortality. The comparison of microscopic craniectomy and endoscopic approach for recurrent or residual pituitary adenomas remains controversial.

Heringer performed a meta-analysis to evaluate effect of repeated trans-sphenoidal surgery in recurrent or residual pituitary adenomas and found that half of secreting tumors and more than half of nonfunctional pituitary adenomas (NFPAs) could achieve remission after surgery, and there is no difference between endoscopic and microscopic approach [6]. However, Esquenazi and his colleagues performed another meta-analysis to compare the effects of endoscopic and microscopic trans-sphenoidal surgery on recurrent and/or residual pituitary adenomas and found that endoscopic surgery led to modest increases in resection rates on residual or recurrent adenomas [7]. Do et al. [8] retrospectively analyzed 61 patients with recurrent or residual pituitary adenomas who underwent endoscopic endonasal surgery and found that the gross total resection was achieved in 31 patients (51.7%), indicating that endoscopic endonasal approach is a safe and effective option for recurrent pituitary adenomas. The results from another meta-analysis performed by Li also indicated that the endoscopic surgery is related to higher gross tumor removal and lower incidence of complications in patients with PA [9]. Almeida accessed the outcomes of reoperation for patients with residual or recurrent growth hormone-secreting PA from authors' institution, and no statistically significant difference was found in disease control rates between the reoperation and first-time neurosurgery. They further systematically reviewed 161 reoperations and 2189 first-time surgery cases retrieved from 29 papers and found that reoperation and first-time surgery had similar control rates for microadenomas, but the reoperation was related to substantially lower control rates for macroadenomas (27.5%) and tumors invading the cavernous sinus (14.7%) [10]. In 2016, a systematic review and evidence-based guideline for the residual or recurrent NFPAs was produced by Congress of Neurological Surgeons, and the repeat resection is recommended as level III recommendations for the treatment of symptomatic recurrent or residual NFPAs [11].

Based on the previous studies and our experience, endoscopic surgery is better than the microscopic surgery for recurrent pituitary adenomas; however, these findings are needed to be verified by the large-scale prospective randomized controlled trials. Therefore, maximum tumor resection, meanwhile preserving nerve function is the goal to achieve local control and decompress vital structures for those refractory PAs with compressive symptoms.

3. Radiation therapy

Despite the success of trans-sphenoidal surgery or maximum tumor resection, most refractory PAs will regrow or recur; therefore, other therapeutic approaches are usually necessary. If surgical and/medical therapy failed to control the tumor growth, radiation therapy (RT) is currently the next treatment option [1]. There are several RT options for patients with refractory PAs. Fractionated external beam radiation therapy (EBRT) has been used for several decades and has shown good clinical safety and efficacy [12]. Stereotactic radiosurgery (SRS) is the delivery of a high single dose of radiation under conditions of accurate positioning. Recently, SRS has been gaining popularity due to the minimizing exposure of normal brain tissue to radiation. SRS has been preferred over fractionated photon beam because of the convenience of single day therapy and the potential for the faster effect on tumor [13]. A variety of SRS including Gamma Knife, CyberKnife, and proton-beam RT are available to deliver stereotactic RT. However, some refractory PAs are not candidates for stereotactic RT because of the tumor size (>3 cm), or tumor location near the optic apparatus and brainstem (<5 mm) [14]. Risks associated with RT include hypopituitarism, optic neuropathy, and other cranial neuropathies, which should be concerned and avoided [12].

Comparing EBRT and SRS may help to guide decision making for patients with residual or recurrent pituitary tumors. Kong et al. [15] compared the efficacy and safety of SRS and EBRT for the treatment of 125 patients with PAs. Although no significant difference was found in either biochemical remission or tumor growth control, the time to biochemical remission after SRS was much shorter than EBRT (26 months vs. 63 months).

To better understand the effects of SRS for Cushing disease (CD), Mehta et al. [16] performed an international, multicenter, retrospective cohort analysis, 278 patients with CD received SRS was retrospective cohort analyzed, and found that the overall rate of durable control of hypercortisolism was 64% for 10 years, and the adverse radiation effects included hypopituitarism (25%) and cranial neuropathy (3%) were observed.

Both conventional radiotherapy and stereotactic RT have shown a good tumoristatic effect on typical PAs; however, they may be largely ineffective and rarely maintain a long-term remission in refractory PAs. As a matter of fact, one of the aggressive PAs with high recurrent potential, silent corticotroph PAs, is with high sensitivity to radiation, so RT can be a good option for patients with those kind of PAs.

4. Medical therapy

Medical therapy plays an increasingly important role in the management of PAs. Temozolomide (TMZ), an orally administered alkylating chemotherapy, is recommended as the first-line chemotherapy for aggressive pituitary tumors and pituitary carcinomas after the failure of standard therapies by the European Society of Endocrinology [17]. TMZ is considered the standard treatment in the management of gliomas. Since 2006, the first successful treatment of PA with TMZ was reported [18, 19], and TMZ treatment has also been widely used for patients with refractory PAs and carcinomas [20]. However, only about 50% of pituitary tumors are sensitive to TMZ treatment, and most of the refractory PAs failed to respond to TMZ and even acquired TMZ resistance after the effective response to TMZ [21]. Therefore, it is important to enhance the efficacy of TMZ and overcome the resistance of TMZ. Some molecular status of pituitary tumors, such as O^6—methylguanine-DNA-methyltransferase MGMT and MSH6, has been associated with temozolomide response [22]. It is reported that the PI3K/AKT/mTOR signaling pathway is upregulated in pituitary tumors, and the inhibition of this pathway may enhance the TMZ-mediated cytotoxicity [23].

Epidermal growth factor receptor (EGFR) is a cell growth factor, which regulates cell proliferation and hormone production in pituitary tumors [24]. EGFR is overexpressed in prolactinoma and ACTH-secreting pituitary adenomas, which may offer a potential therapeutic target for refractory pituitary tumors [25, 26]. As an EGFR inhibitor, gefitinib has shown antiproliferative and apoptotic effects in corticotroph tumor cell *in vitro* [25]. Lapatinib, a dual HER2/EGFR inhibitor, was shown to both suppressed PRL mRNA expression and secretion more than gefitinib in animal model of prolactinomas [27].

Although further clinical trials are needed, preclinical data suggest that the EGFR pathway may be an effective therapeutic targeting for patients with refractory pituitary tumors.

Vascular endothelial growth factor (VEGF) is a potent angiogenic factor in pituitary tumors. The previous studies indicated that angiogenesis is associated with adenoma development, local invasion, and recurrences [28–30]. Several researches reported that angiogenesis decrease tumor sizes in human and experimental pituitary tumors [31–33]. Ortiz has reported the first case of a bevacizumab-treated pituitary carcinoma with long-term stabilization of disease in 2012 [34]. Touma also presented one case of pituitary carcinoma treated successfully with concurrent chemoradiation therapy and bevacizumab with a long-term follow up [35]. However, the role of anti-VEGF therapy in pituitary tumors is still controversial due to the lack of large-scale clinical trial.

Phosphatidylinositol 3-kinase (PI3K)/AKT/mammalian target of rapamycin (mTOR) cascades is key signaling pathways in tumorigenesis of pituitary adenoma [36]. The previous studies reported that the PI3K/AKT/mTOR pathway is upregulated and overactivated in pituitary adenomas, implicating an important role in tumor formation and progression of pituitary adenoma [37–39]. Inhibition of the PI3K/mTOR signaling pathway not only displays antitumor efficacy against pituitary tumor [40, 41] but also sensitizes pituitary adenoma cells to radiotherapy and chemotherapy [23, 42]. Donovan reported one patient with pituitary carcinoma, which is refractory to multiple surgery, radiation, and chemotherapy, after the treatment with mTOR inhibitor (everolimus) and radiation, and the clinical improvement and stability >6 months were achieved [43].

As a promising therapeutic approach, cancer immunotherapy has been attracting more and more attention recently. To date, immunotherapy has been applied for the treatment of many tumors including glioma, lung cancer, melanoma, prostate cancer, and B cell lymphoma [44]. In 2007, Hazrati and his colleagues have reported one case of a prolactinoma treated successfully with immunotherapy for the first time [45]. Lu has reported that CD68+ macrophage infiltration is associated with the pituitary adenoma size and invasiveness, indicating that immunotherapy may be useful to restrict the tumor enlargement and invasiveness [46]. Blocking the interaction between the programmed cell death (PD-1) protein and one of its ligands, programmed death ligand 1 (PD-L1) is one of the novel strategies for cancer immunotherapy. The expression of PD-L1 is positively correlated with improved responses to anti-PD-1/PD-L1 blockade in many cancers [47]. Mei reported that the expression of (PD-L1) is significantly higher in human functioning adenomas compared to nonfunctioning adenomas, suggesting the existence of an immune response to pituitary tumors [48]. Therefore, these researches raise the possibility of considering immunotherapy for the refractory PAs.

5. Conclusion

Although various treatment options are available to manage these refractory pituitary tumors, the efficacy is limited. Therefore, the new therapeutic approaches and such randomized clinical trials are needed. It is hoped that further research may clarify the tumorigenesis and pathogenesis of refractory PAs, and additional alternative treatments may be developed for these tumors in the near future.

Declaration of interest

None of the authors have potential financial conflicts of interests related to this article. The financial support for this study was provided by the National Natural Science Foundation of China (grant number: 81502639, 81501192), Scientific Research Project of Capital Health Development in 2018 (grant number: 2018-4-4018), and the Youth Scientific Research Fund in Peking Union Medical College Hospital (grant number: pumch-2016-2.20). The funding institutions had no role in the design of the study, data collection and analysis, the decision to publish, or the preparation of the manuscript.

Abbreviations

TMZ	temozolomide
WHO	World health organization
IHC	immunohistochemical stain
ACTH	adrenocorticotropic hormone
CD	Cushing disease
CS	Cushing's syndrome
DA	dopamine agonists
EBRT	external beam radiation therapy
EGFR	epidermal growth factor receptor
NFPA	nonfunctional pituitary adenomas
PD-L1	programmed death ligand 1
RPA	refractory pituitary adenoma
RT	radiation therapy
SRS	stereotactic radiosurgery
TSS	trans-sphenoidal surgery
VEGF	vascular endothelial growth factor

Author details

Congxin Dai[1], Xiaohai Liu[1], Sihai Ma[1], Ming Feng[1], Xinjie Bao[1], Kan Deng[1], Yong Yao[1], Renzhi Wang[1*], DX. Feng[2], E. Fonkem[2], Frank Y. Shan[2] and Jason H. Huang[2]

1 Department of Neurosurgery, Peking Union Medical College Hospital, Chinese Academy of Medical Sciences and Peking Union Medical College, Beijing, P.R. China

2 Department of Neurosurgery, Ballor Scott and White Medical Center, College of Medicine, Texas A&M University, Temple, TX, USA

*Address all correspondence to: wangrz@126.com

IntechOpen

© 2018 The Author(s). Licensee IntechOpen. This chapter is distributed under the terms of the Creative Commons Attribution License (http://creativecommons.org/licenses/by/3.0), which permits unrestricted use, distribution, and reproduction in any medium, provided the original work is properly cited.

References

[1] Colao A, Grasso LF, Pivonello R, Lombardi G. Therapy of aggressive pituitary tumors. Expert Opinion on Pharmacotherapy. 2011;**12**(10): 1561-1570

[2] Dai C, Feng M, Liu X, Ma S, Sun B, Bao X, et al. Refractory pituitary adenoma: A novel classification for pituitary tumors. Oncotarget. 2016; 7(50):83657-83668

[3] Chatzellis E, Alexandraki KI, Androulakis II, Kaltsas G. Aggressive pituitary tumors. Neuroendocrinology. 2015;**101**(2):87-104

[4] Heaney A. Management of aggressive pituitary adenomas and pituitary carcinomas. Journal of Neuro-Oncology. 2014;**117**(3):459-468

[5] Hirohata T, Ishii Y, Matsuno A. Treatment of pituitary carcinomas and atypical pituitary adenomas: A review. Neurologia Medico-Chirurgica. 2014; **54**(12):966-973

[6] Heringer LC, de Oliveira MF, Rotta JM, Botelho RV. Effect of repeated transsphenoidal surgery in recurrent or residual pituitary adenomas: A systematic review and meta-analysis. Surgical Neurology International. 2016; **7**:14

[7] Esquenazi Y, Essayed WI, Singh H, Mauer E, Ahmed M, Christos PJ, et al. Endoscopic endonasal versus microscopic transsphenoidal surgery for recurrent and/or residual pituitary adenomas. World Neurosurgery. 2017; **101**:186-195

[8] Do H, Kshettry VR, Siu A, Belinsky I, Farrell CJ, Nyquist G, et al. Extent of resection, visual, and endocrinologic outcomes for endoscopic endonasal surgery for recurrent pituitary adenomas. World Neurosurgery. 2017; **102**:35-41

[9] Li A, Liu W, Cao P, Zheng Y, Bu Z, Zhou T. Endoscopic versus microscopic transsphenoidal surgery in the treatment of pituitary adenoma: A systematic review and meta-analysis. World Neurosurgery. 2017;**101**:236-246

[10] Almeida JP, Ruiz-Trevino AS, Liang B, Omay SB, Shetty SR, Chen YN, et al. Reoperation for growth hormone-secreting pituitary adenomas: Report on an endonasal endoscopic series with a systematic review and meta-analysis of the literature. Journal of Neurosurgery; **2017**:1-13

[11] Rughani A, Schwalb JM, Sidiropoulos C, Pilitsis J, Ramirez-Zamora A, Sweet JA, et al. Congress of neurological surgeons systematic review and evidence-based guideline on subthalamic nucleus and globus pallidus internus deep brain stimulation for the treatment of patients with Parkinson's disease: Executive summary. Neurosurgery. 2018;**82**(6):753-756

[12] Tritos NA, Biller BMK. Update on radiation therapy in patients with Cushing's disease. Pituitary. 2015;**18**(2): 263-268

[13] Lee C, Sheehan JP. Advances in Gamma Knife radiosurgery for pituitary tumors. Current Opinion in Endocrinology, Diabetes, and Obesity. 2016;**23**(4):331-338

[14] Buchfelder M. Management of aggressive pituitary adenomas: Current treatment strategies. Pituitary. 2009; **12**(3):256-260

[15] Kong D, Lee J, Lim DH, Kim KW, Shin HJ, Nam D, et al. The efficacy of fractionated radiotherapy and stereotactic radiosurgery for pituitary

adenomas. Cancer. 2007;**110**(4): 854-860

[16] Mehta GU, Ding D, Patibandla MR, Kano H, Sisterson N, Su YH, et al. Stereotactic radiosurgery for cushing disease: Results of an international, multicenter study. The Journal of Clinical Endocrinology and Metabolism. 2017;**102**(11):4284-4291

[17] Raverot G, Burman P, McCormack A, Heaney A, Petersenn S, Popovic V, et al. European Society of Endocrinology Clinical Practice Guidelines for the management of aggressive pituitary tumours and carcinomas. European Journal of Endocrinology. 2018;**178**(1): G1-G24

[18] Fadul CE, Kominsky AL, Meyer LP, Kingman LS, Kinlaw WB, Rhodes CH, et al. Long-term response of pituitary carcinoma to temozolomide. Report of two cases. Journal of Neurosurgery. 2006;**105**(4):621-626

[19] Lim S, Shahinian H, Maya MM, Yong W, Heaney AP. Temozolomide: A novel treatment for pituitary carcinoma. The Lancet Oncology. 2006;**7**(6): 518-520

[20] Losa M, Bogazzi F, Cannavo S, Ceccato F, Curt L, De Marinis L, et al. Temozolomide therapy in patients with aggressive pituitary adenomas or carcinomas. Journal of Neuro-Oncology. 2016;**126**(3):519-525

[21] Lasolle H, Cortet C, Castinetti F, Cloix L, Caron P, Delemer B, et al. Temozolomide treatment can improve overall survival in aggressive pituitary tumors and pituitary carcinomas. European Journal of Endocrinology. 2017;**176**(6):769-777

[22] Matsuno A, Murakami M, Hoya K, Yamada SM, Miyamoto S, Yamada S, et al. Molecular status of pituitary carcinoma and atypical adenoma that contributes the effectiveness of temozolomide. Medical Molecular Morphology. 2014;**47**(1):1-7

[23] Dai C, Zhang B, Liu X, Ma S, Yang Y, Yao Y, et al. Inhibition of PI3K/AKT/mTOR pathway enhances temozolomide-induced cytotoxicity in pituitary adenoma cell lines in vitro and xenografted pituitary adenoma in female nude mice. Endocrinology. 2013; **154**(3):1247-1259

[24] Cooper O, Mamelak A, Bannykh S, Carmichael J, Bonert V, Lim S, et al. Prolactinoma ErbB receptor expression and targeted therapy for aggressive tumors. Endocrine. 2014;**46**(2):318-327

[25] Fukuoka H, Cooper O, Ben-Shlomo A, Mamelak A, Ren S, Bruyette D, et al. EGFR as a therapeutic target for human, canine, and mouse ACTH-secreting pituitary adenomas. The Journal of Clinical Investigation. 2011;**121**(12): 4712-4721

[26] Fukuoka H, Cooper O, Mizutani J, Tong Y, Ren SG, Bannykh S, et al. HER2/ErbB2 receptor signaling in rat and human prolactinoma cells: Strategy for targeted prolactinoma therapy. Molecular Endocrinology. 2011;**25**(1): 92-103

[27] Liu X, Kano M, Araki T, Cooper O, Fukuoka H, Tone Y, et al. ErbB receptor-driven prolactinomas respond to targeted lapatinib treatment in female transgenic mice. Endocrinology. 2015; **156**(1):71-79

[28] Cristina C, Luque GM, Demarchi G, Lopez Vicchi F, Zubeldia-Brenner L, Perez Millan MI, et al. Angiogenesis in pituitary adenomas: human studies and new mutant mouse models. International Journal of Endocrinology. 2014;**2014**:608497

[29] Sánchez-Ortiga R, Sánchez-Tejada L, Moreno-Perez O, Riesgo P, Niveiro M, Picó Alfonso AM. Over-expression of vascular endothelial growth factor in

pituitary adenomas is associated with extrasellar growth and recurrence. Pituitary. 2013;**16**(3):370-377

[30] Jia W, Sander AJ, Jia G, Ni M, Liu X, Lu R, et al. Vascular endothelial growth inhibitor (VEGI) is an independent indicator for invasion in human pituitary adenomas. Anticancer Research. 2013;**33**(9):3815-3822

[31] Lee KM, Park SH, Park KS, Hwang JH, Hwang SK. Analysis of circulating endostatin and vascular endothelial growth factor in patients with pituitary adenoma treated by stereotactic radiosurgery: A Preliminary Study. Brain Tumor Research and Treatment. 2015;**3**(2):89-94

[32] Miyajima K, Takekoshi S, Itoh J, Kakimoto K, Miyakoshi T, Osamura RY. Inhibitory effects of anti-VEGF antibody on the growth and angiogenesis of estrogen-induced pituitary prolactinoma in fischer 344 rats: Animal model of VEGF-targeted therapy for human endocrine tumors. Acta Histochemica et Cytochemica. 2010;**43**(2):33-44

[33] Cohen AB, Lessell S. Angiogenesis and pituitary tumors. Seminars in Ophthalmology. 2009;**24**(3):185-189

[34] Ortiz LD, Syro LV, Scheithauer BW, Ersen A, Uribe H, Fadul CE, et al. Anti-VEGF therapy in pituitary carcinoma. Pituitary. 2012;**15**(3):445-449

[35] Touma W, Hoostal S, Peterson RA, Wiernik A, SantaCruz KS, Lou E. Successful treatment of pituitary carcinoma with concurrent radiation, temozolomide, and bevacizumab after resection. Journal of Clinical Neuroscience. 2017;**41**:75-77

[36] Dworakowska D, Wlodek E, Leontiou CA, Igreja S, Cakir M, Teng M, et al. Activation of RAF/MEK/ERK and PI3K/AKT/mTOR pathways in pituitary adenomas and their effects on downstream effectors. Endocrine-Related Cancer. 2009;**16**(4): 1329-1338

[37] Sajjad EA, Zielinski G, Maksymowicz M, Hutnik L, Bednarczuk T, Wlodarski P. mTOR is frequently active in GH-secreting pituitary adenomas without influencing their morphopathological features. Endocrine Pathology. 2013;**24**(1):11-19

[38] Rubinfeld H, Shimon I. PI3K/Akt/mTOR and Raf/MEK/ERK signaling pathways perturbations in non-functioning pituitary adenomas. Endocrine. 2012;**42**(2):285-291

[39] Chen R, Duan J, Li L, Ma Q, Sun Q, Ma J, et al. mTOR promotes pituitary tumor development through activation of PTTG1. Oncogene. 2017;**36**(7): 979-988

[40] Monsalves E, Juraschka K, Tateno T, Agnihotri S, Asa SL, Ezzat S, et al. The PI3K/AKT/mTOR pathway in the pathophysiology and treatment of pituitary adenomas. Endocrine-Related Cancer. 2014;**21**(4):R331-R344

[41] Lee M, Wiedemann T, Gross C, Leinhauser I, Roncaroli F, Braren R, et al. Targeting PI3K/mTOR signaling displays potent antitumor efficacy against nonfunctioning pituitary adenomas. Clinical Cancer Research. 2015;**21**(14):3204-3215

[42] Sukumari-Ramesh S, Singh N, Dhandapani KM, Vender JR. mTOR inhibition reduces cellular proliferation and sensitizes pituitary adenoma cells to ionizing radiation. Surgical Neurology International. 2011;**2**:22

[43] Donovan LE, Arnal AV, Wang SH, Odia Y. Widely metastatic atypical pituitary adenoma with mTOR pathway STK11(F298L) mutation treated with everolimus therapy. CNS Oncology. 2016;**5**(4):203-209

[44] Grullich C. Immunotherapy as modern tumor treatment. Radiologe. 2017;**57**(10):822-825

[45] Hazrati SM, Aghazadeh J, Mohtarami F, Abouzari M, Rashidi A. Immunotherapy of prolactinoma with a T helper 1 activator adjuvant and autoantigens: A case report. Neuroimmunomodulation. 2007;**13**(4): 205-208

[46] Lu J, Adam B, Jack AS, Lam A, Broad RW, Chik CL. Immune cell infiltrates in pituitary adenomas: More macrophages in larger adenomas and more T cells in growth hormone adenomas. Endocrine Pathology. 2015; **26**(3):263-272

[47] Topalian SL, Hodi FS, Brahmer JR, Gettinger SN, Smith DC, McDermott DF, et al. Safety, activity, and immune correlates of anti-PD-1 antibody in cancer. The New England Journal of Medicine. 2012;**366**(26):2443-2454

[48] Mei Y, Bi WL, Greenwald NF, Du Z, Agar NY, Kaiser UB, et al. Increased expression of programmed death ligand 1 (PD-L1) in human pituitary tumors. Oncotarget. 2016;**7**(47):76565-76576

Chapter 6

Vestibular Schwannomas: Diagnosis and Surgical Treatment

Gustavo Jung and Ricardo Ramina

Abstract

Over the last decades, significant advances in skull base surgery have enabled many neurosurgical centers around the world to perform surgical resection of vestibular schwannomas; otherwise, clinical observation and radiotherapy/radiosurgery can be possible management options. Auditory pattern, the presence of bilateral tumors, tumor size, and neurological symptoms are deeply considered in the decision-making process. In this chapter, we expanded the general discussion of vestibular schwannomas, discussing bases for an accurate diagnose and the technical aspects for the surgical approaches, drilling of internal auditory canal, and its reconstruction as well as the technical nuances when handling very small and large/residual tumors.

Keywords: vestibular schwannoma, acoustic neuroma, acoustic tumor, cerebellopontine angle

1. Introduction

Vestibular schwannomas (VS) account for 6–8% of all intracranial neoplasms and around 90% of cerebellopontine angle tumors (CPA) [1]. It is usually a sporadic tumor but can be bilateral in cases of neurofibromatosis type 2, when larger tumors are common.

Over the last decades, significant advances in skull base surgery have enabled many neurosurgical centers around the world to perform surgical resection of VS with good functional outcomes (facial nerve and hearing preservation). Deeper observation about the natural history of these lesions and the development of radiosurgery have increased the options to manage VS. The rates of surgical morbidity and mortality have also declined dramatically, and functional preservation of the facial nerve has been possible even in larger tumors.

2. Natural history

The natural history of VS is highly unpredictable. Some tumors exhibit continuous growth, while others remain stable or even decrease in size, and its reason is not known. In the literature, a mean growth rate of 2.9 mm per year is reported, and a growth rate of 2.5 mm/year is associated with worse hearing function.

IntechOpen

3. Management options

Clinical observation, microsurgical removal, and radiotherapy/radiosurgery are the management options. Different factors make treatment decision highly variable. Small tumors may be followed with regular MRI examinations and audiograms. Patients harboring small tumors and presenting progressive hearing loss, microsurgical removal, or radiosurgery should be considered. Preoperative hearing level is a prognostic factor for postoperative hearing preservation. Tumors up to 3 cm in diameter may be treated either by microsurgical removal or radiosurgery, and larger tumors will require surgical resection. Cystic VS may present sudden growth and surgical removal is the best option. The management of bilateral tumors in NF2 patients is complex, and the quality of hearing in both ears and size of the tumors will be the main factors to decide how to treat these patients.

4. Diagnosis

VS commonly arise from the vestibular division of the eighth cranial nerve. Dizziness, vertigo, and progressive hearing loss (earliest symptom) are the most frequent complaints. Dizziness is routinely transient and episodic, and the patient can neglect it for a variable period of time. Dizziness is a frequent complaint in daily ENT practice, and patients complaining of unilateral hearing loss associated or not to vestibular symptoms are frequently seen by ENT surgeons. Very often these symptoms are not adequately investigated, and it is a common cause to miss the diagnosis.

Facial nerve weakness is observed in only 6% of the patients [2]. In larger and mainly cystic tumors that present fast growth, facial numbness (due to trigeminal nerve compression) and gait ataxia (due to brain stem displacement) can appear [3, 4].

Hydrocephalus is relatively common in VS patients. In larger tumors it is caused by IV ventricle displacement, leading to obstructive hydrocephalus. In smaller tumors, degenerative changes on the tumor content can increase the protein rates on CSF, causing CSF malabsorption and consequent hydrocephalus [5]. When hydrocephalus is present, a preoperative external ventricular CSF drainage is required. Ventriculoperitoneal shunt is done especially in patients without major CSF obstruction when the tumor removal is less probable to relieve.

5. Audiological evaluation

Hearing function is evaluated with audiograms with sound discrimination. There are different classifications to preoperatively grade the hearing function. Brain stem evoked response audiometry (BERA) provides reliable information on the hearing function from the ear to the brain stem, and to determine the nerve of origin in vestibular schwannomas, the video Head Impulse Test (vHIT) is usually performed.

6. Radiological diagnosis

CT scan is useful to demonstrate the bony anatomy, the position of the jugular bulb, and the semicircular canals. Vestibular schwannomas often expand the internal auditory canal [10].

DOI: http://dx.doi.org/10.5772/intechopen.81352

Magnetic resonance imaging (MRI) is the eligible test to diagnose and evaluate patients with a vestibular schwannomas. T1, T2, FLAIR, and DWI images are usually sufficient for the diagnosis. Over 50% of vestibular schwannomas are isointense in T1-weighted images; hypointensities usually represent a cystic component (**Figure 1**). VS present usually intense homogeneous gadolinium enhancement on T1-weighted images, but cystic lesions can present a heterogenous pattern. A hyperintense signal inside of the IAC in FLAIR images and nodular hyperintense signal in the vestibular nuclei on the dorsal pons in T2-weighted images can additionally differentiate vestibular schwannomas from other cerebellopontine angle tumors (**Figure 2**). T2-weighted images and tractography may demonstrate the position of the facial nerve and its relation to the tumor capsule [5, 6]. When a watchful waiting is decided, MRI volumetric studies have an excellent accuracy to follow tumor growth [7]. 3D T2 CISS or post-contrast 3D T1 MPRAGE MRI (evidence class II) provides best images to monitor tumor growth [8, 9].

After surgical resection, a thin not-nodular enhancement is often visualized in surgical resection field. It can persist for years but usually reduces over the time [11]. Fat grafts, fibrin glue, and muscle grafts, used to reconstruct the IAC, can generate a nodular enhancement which usually appear within the first 3 days after surgery. New nodular enhancement appearing in the postoperative follow-up highly suggests tumor recurrence [12].

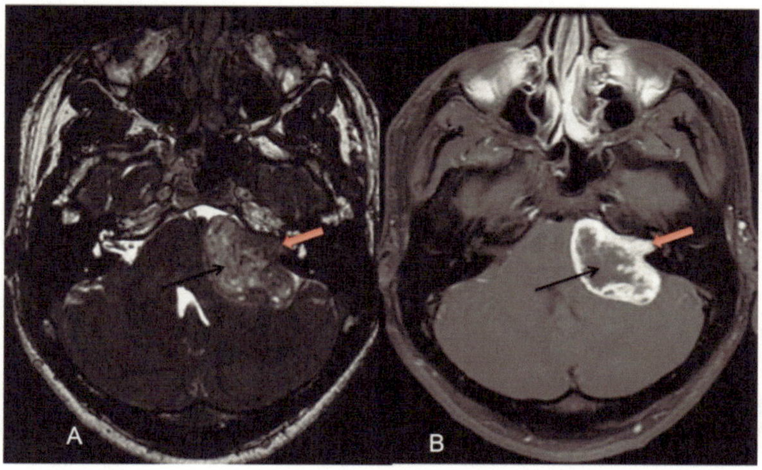

Figure 1.
Large vestibular schwannoma. (A) T2-weighted image showing a solid (red arrow) and cystic tumor (black arrow). (B) Post-contrast-weighted image exhibiting intense contrast enhancement in the solid portion (red arrow) and heterogeneous pattern in the cystic component (black arrow).

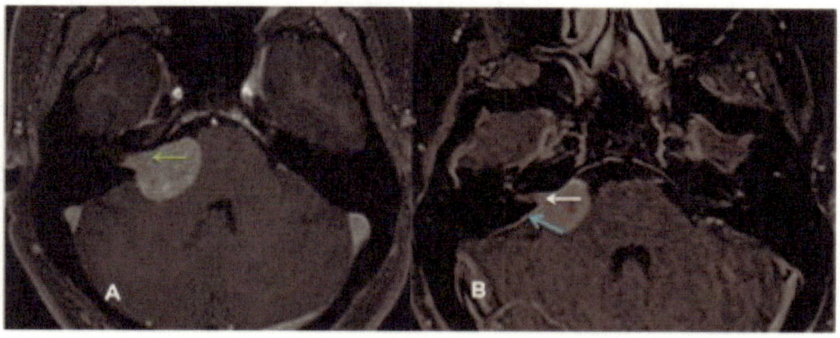

Figure 2.
T2-weighted image with a small vestibular schwannoma (green arrow) with hyperintensity in the dorsal pons (blue arrow).

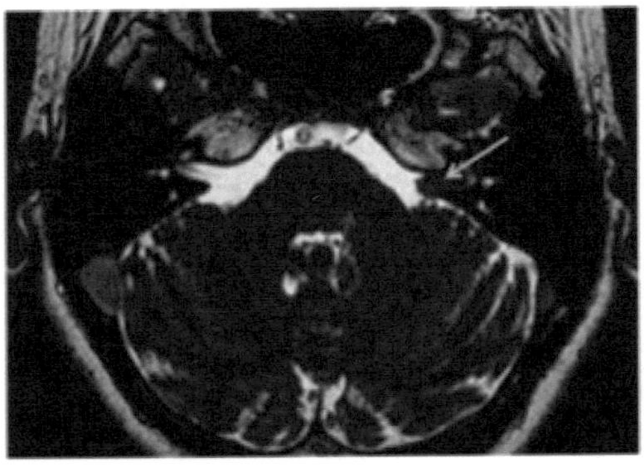

Figure 3.
(A) Expansion of IAC caused by vestibular schwannoma (green arrow). (B) Normal width of IAC in a patient with CPA meningioma and IAC involvement (white arrow). Dural enhancement (blue arrow) strongly suggests its diagnosis.

Meningiomas are the most frequent differential diagnosis between non-schwannomatous lesions that arise or protrude into the IAC. Meningiomas usually present a dural enhancement and display calcification, and hyperostosis in the adjacent bone is usually seen (**Figure 3**).

7. Treatment

Vestibular schwannoma is a benign intracranial nerve sheath tumor, usually sporadic but that may be bilateral in the context of neurofibromatosis type 2. Wait and scan strategy, microsurgical resection, and radiotherapy/radiosurgery are the options. Presenting symptoms, hearing status, growth rate, size and characteristic of tumor, and surgeon preference will interfere in these treatment decisions [13].

8. Microsurgical resection

The goals of the treatment are radical resection with zero mortality and complete anatomical and functional preservation of the involved cranial nerves. Some authors propose partial resection followed, or not, by radiotherapy/radiosurgery to preserve cranial nerve function [14]. However, the only treatment that offers cure is radical microsurgical removal.

VS might be approached through translabyrinthine, retrosigmoid, or middle fossa craniotomy. The main advantage of the translabyrinthine approach is to minimize brain retraction. The difficulty to resect larger tumor damage to hearing structures is the limitation of this surgical approach. Fat grafts are needed to close the dura and avoid CSF fistula. In small tumors, best suited to tranlabyrinthine approach, commonly serviceable hearing is present, which ultimately turns this surgical option unfeasible.

The middle fossa approach (MFA) is a lateral access to the IAC and was popularized by House in 1961. The exposition of the IAC through its superior wall makes it a good option for small lateral tumors restricted to the internal auditory canal and brings the lowest risk to the labyrinth structures.

The retrosigmoid (RS) approach is the most used access by the majority of neurosurgeons offering an excellent exposition of all anatomical structures of the posterior fossa. The IAC is opened through the RS, and injury to the inner ear structures (labyrinth) and jugular bulb are avoidable complications [15]. This is the approach of choice to VS, regardless of its size, in our department. The dorsal decubitus is preferred by the authors due to the lower risk of air embolism and to provide a more comfortable work position for the surgeon.

A 4 cm diameter craniotomy is cut laterally bordering the sigmoid sinus to avoid cerebellar retraction. In most cases, in the dorsal position, a cerebellar retractor is only used to protect the cerebellum during the drilling of internal auditory canal.

After the dura opening, CSF is released from the cerebellomedullary cisterna to relax the pressure in the posterior fossa. The inspection of the bridging veins over the tentorial surface of the cerebellum is highly recommended as it can be a potential source of bleeding.

The IAC is drilled as the first step in most cases. It reduces the pressure over the cochlear and the facial nerves. Piecemeal resection with ultrasound aspirator is useful to debulk the cisternal component and reduces the traction over the tumor capsule. The facial nerve is usually very attached to the tumor capsule at its entrance in the IAC, and careful microsurgical dissection should be performed under continuous electrophysiologic monitoring. Preservation of the cochlear nerve is also attempted under continuous BERA monitoring. If an alteration of the waves is observed, the surgical field is irrigated with papaverine solution awaiting until recovery is recorded. Cystic and larger tumors usually present more difficulty to dissect the facial nerve from tumor capsule. Hearing preservation is a challenge in tumors larger than 3 cm in diameter. In NF2 patients with bilateral tumor, preservation of hearing should be attempted even if residual tumor must be left. Brain stem decompression with hearing preservation is the goal of treatment in these cases.

Reconstruction of the IAC is extremely important to avoid CSF fistula and infection. To identify the mastoid air cells inside the IAC, the use of the endoscope can be opportune, and small pieces of muscle or fat graft should be used to seal these cells.

9. Residual tumor

In our series of 541 VS surgically resected between 1987 and 2016, 31 patients had residual/recurrent tumors. Twenty-seven patients had been operated elsewhere. From the 4 patients in our own casuistry, two cases were recurrences and two were residual lesions. One of the residual cases was a patient with neurofibromatosis type 2 and showing large bilateral VS who underwent radical resection in one side and subtotal removal of the contralateral tumor for hearing preservation. The other case was a 75-year-old patient with large cystic VS who underwent stereotactic aspiration of the cyst to alleviate mass effect, since surgical resection was not advised for medical reasons.

The causes for subtotal removal, as reported by the patient, were extensive intraoperative bleeding, adherence to the brain stem or facial nerve, and intraoperative cerebellar edema. All patients were reoperated at our institution through the retrosigmoid/transmeatal approach. The surgical procedure proved to be significantly more difficult than in non-operated cases. Fibrosis from previous procedure(s) altered the anatomical location of the transverse and sigmoid sinus, as well as the dissection and opening of the dura mater. Intracranially, the arachnoid plane usually found between the tumor and the brain stem and cranial nerves was lost; thus, dissection of the tumor required more manipulation of those structures. This was especially significant in irradiated patients. We observed that in cases in which the IAC had not been previously opened, identification and dissection of the facial nerve and subsequent dissection were less difficult. Postoperative anatomical preservation of the facial nerve was possible in 13 (76%) of 17 patients with preoperative facial nerve function. There was no permanent morbidity or mortality. All cases were histologically confirmed as WHO grade I schwannomas [16].

10. Intralabyrinthine tumors

Intralabyrinthine VS are by definition tumors arising at the terminal end of the eighth cranial nerve within the vestibule, cochlea, or semicircular canal [17]. According to its location, intralabyrinthine schwannomas may be anatomically divided in six major types: intravestibular, vestibulocochlear, modiolar, transotic, intracochlear, and transmacular schwannomas (**Figures 4–7**).

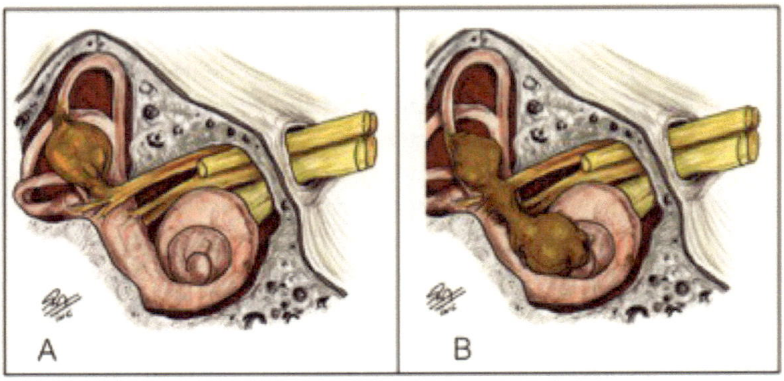

Figure 4.
(A) Intravestibular schwannoma. (B) Vestibulocochlear schwannoma. Intravestibular schwannomas are located in the labyrinth. Vestibulocochlear schwannomas grow in the labyrinth and cochlea.

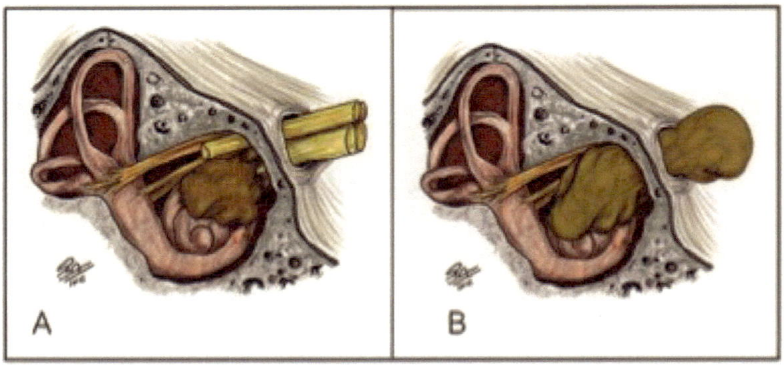

Figure 5.
(A) Modiolar schwannoma. (B) Transotic schwannoma.

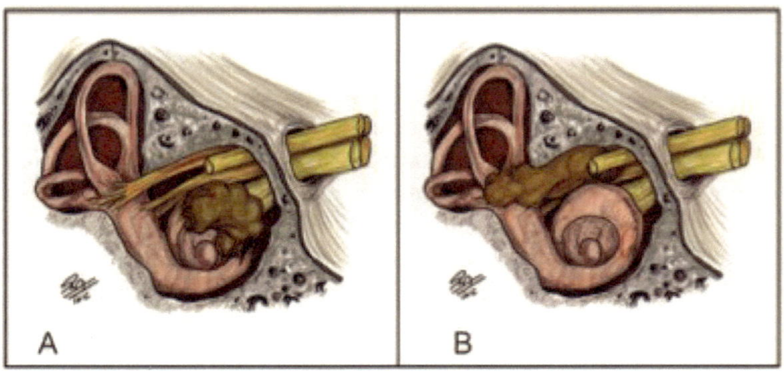

Figure 6.
(A) Intracochlear schwannoma. (B) Transmacular schwannoma.

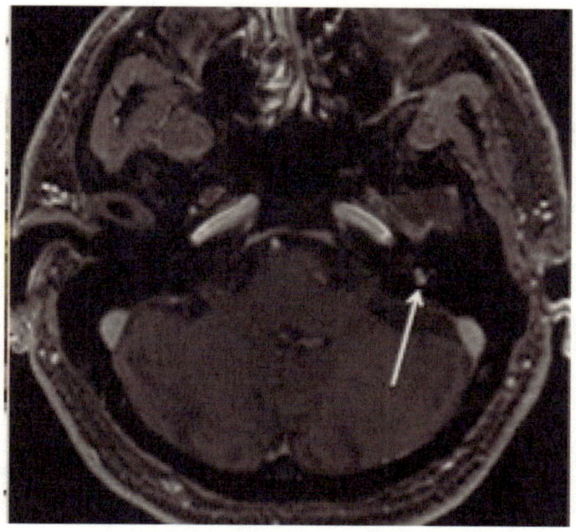

Figure 7.
Post-contrast T1-weighted image demonstrating a transmacular schwannoma (white arrow).

Modiolar schwannomas arise at the cochlea and extend in the modiolus and the IAC. Transotic schwannomas grow from the labyrinth into the IAC and middle ear.

Intracochlear schwannomas are located in the cochlea. Transmacular schwannomas arise in the vestibule and extend into the internal auditory canal through the macula cribrosa.

These tumors have been frequently observed on MRI examinations, but their management was rarely reported in the literature [18].

Labyrinthitis and otitis may also cause gadolinium enhancement of the vestibular nerves and mimic intralabyrinthine tumors. However, in these pathologies the enhancement is less sharp, and the cochlea, as well as the entire vestibular system, may exhibit contrast enhancement [19].

Clinical observation is recommended in patients already deaf and if the vestibular symptoms are slight and treatable. Microsurgical removal is curative, but hearing preservation is very challenging since these tumors often affect the cochlea and the semicircular canals. The retrosigmoid-transmeatal endoscopic-assisted approach is very useful and provides an excellent view of the lateral portion of IAC. A wide and deep opening of the IAC (about 1 cm in length) is required to resect those lesions. Symptoms of intractable vertigo usually disappear after microsurgical removal of the lesion [20, 21].

Author details

Gustavo Jung* and Ricardo Ramina
Skull Base Division, Department of Neurosurgery, Neurological Institute of Curitiba, Curitiba, Brazil

*Address all correspondence to: gustavosjung@gmail.com

IntechOpen

© 2019 The Author(s). Licensee IntechOpen. This chapter is distributed under the terms of the Creative Commons Attribution License (http://creativecommons.org/licenses/by/3.0), which permits unrestricted use, distribution, and reproduction in any medium, provided the original work is properly cited.

References

[1] Machinis TG, Fountas KN, Dimomopolos V, Robinson JS. History of acoustic neurinoma surgery. Neurosurgical Focus. 2005;**18**(4):1-4

[2] Matthies C, Samii M. Management of 1000 vestibular schwannomas (acoustic neuromas): Clinical presentation. Neurosurgery. 1997;**40**(1):1-10

[3] Piccirillo E, Wiet MR, Flanagan S, Dispenza F, Giannuzzi A, Mancini F, et al. Cystic vestibular schwannoma: Classification, management, and facial nerve outcomes. Otology & Neurotology. 2009;**30**(6):826-834

[4] Thakur JD, Khan IS, Shorter CD, Sonig A, Gardner GL, Guthikonda B, et al. Do cystic vestibular schwannomas have worse surgical outcomes: Systematic analysis of the literature. Neurosurgical Focus. 2012;**33**(3):E12

[5] Taniguchi M, Nakai T, Kohta M, Kimura H, Kohmura E. Communicating hydrocephalus associated with small- to medium-sized vestibular schwannomas: Clinical significance of the tumor apparent diffusion coefficient map. World Neurosurgery. 2016;**94**:261-267

[6] Liang C, Zhang B, Wu L, Du Y, Wang X, Liu C, et al. The superiority of 3D-CISS sequence in displaying the cisternal segment of facial, vestibulocochlear nerves and their abnormal changes. European Journal of Radiology. 2010;**74**(3):437-440

[7] Choi KS, Kim MS, Kwon HG, Jang SH, Kim OL. Preoperative identification of facial nerve in vestibular schwannomas surgery using diffusion tensor tractography. Journal of Korean Neurosurgical Association. 2014;**56**(1):11-15

[8] Tan TY. Non-contrast high resolution fast spin echo magnetic resonance imaging of acoustic schwannoma. Singapore Medical Journal. 1999;**40**(1):27-31

[9] Held P, Fellner C, Seitz J, Graf S, Fellner F, Strutz J. The value of T2(*)-weighted MR images for the diagnosis of acoustic neuromas. European Journal of Radiology. 1999;**30**(3):237-244

[10] Held P, Fellner C, Fellner F, Seitz J, Graf S, Hilbert M, et al. MRI of inner ear and facial nerve pathology using 3D MP-RAGE and 3D CISS sequences. The British Journal of Radiology. 1997;**70**(834):558-566

[11] Tomogane Y, Mori K, Izumoto S, Kaba K, Ishikura R, Ando K, et al. Usefulness of PRESTO magnetic resonance imaging for the differentiation of schwannoma and meningioma in the cerebellopontine angle. Neurologia Medico-Chirurgica (Tokyo). 2013;**53**(7):482-489

[12] Carlson ML, Van Abel KM, Driscoll CL, Neff BA, Beatty CW, Lane JI, et al. Magnetic resonance imaging surveillance following vestibular schwannoma resection. Laryngoscope. 2012;**122**(2):378-388

[13] Bennett ML, Jackson CG, Kaufmann R, Warren F. Postoperative imaging of vestibular schwannomas. Otolaryngology and Head and Neck Surgery. 2008;**138**(5):667-671

[14] Taylor RL, Kong J, Flanagan S, Pogson J, Croxson G, Pohl D, et al. Prevalence of vestibular dysfunction in patients with vestibular schwannoma using video head-impulses and vestibular-evoked potentials. Journal of Neurology. 2015;**262**(5):1228-1237

[15] Samii M, Gerganov VM, Samii A. Functional outcome after complete surgical removal of giant vestibular

schwannomas. Journal of Neurosurgery. 2010;**112**(4):860-867

[16] Tatagiba M, Samii M, Matthies C, El Azm M, Schönmayr R. The significance for postoperative heating of preserving the labyrinth in acoustic neurinoma surgery. Journal of Neurosurgery. 1992;**77**(5):677-684

[17] Kennedy RJ, Shelton C, Salzman KL, Davidson HC, Harnsberger HR. Intralabyrinthine schwannomas: Diagnosis, management, and a new classification system. Otology & Neurotology. 2004;**25**(2):160-167

[18] Magliulo G, Colicchio G, Romana AF, Stasolla A. Intracochlear schwannoma. Skull Base. 2010;**20**(2):115-118

[19] Harnsberger R, Glastonbury CM, Michel MA, Harnsberger HR, Glastonbury CM, Michel MA, et al. Diagnostic Imaging: Head and Neck. 2nd ed. Baltimore: Lippincott, Williams & Wilkins; 2010. https://www.amazon.co.uk/s/ref=dp_byline_sr_book_4?ie=UTF8&text=Bernadette+L.+Koch&search-alias=books-uk&field-author=Bernadette+L.+Koch&sort=relevancerank

[20] Samii M, Matthies C, Tatagiba M. Intracanalicular acoustic neurinomas. Neurosurgery. 1991;**29**(2):189-199

[21] Samii M, Metwali H, Gerganov V. Eficacy of microsurgical tumor removal for treatment of patients with intracanalicular vestibular schwannoma presenting with disabling vestibular symptoms. Journal of Neurosurgery. 2017;**126**(5):1514-1519

Chapter 7

The Systemic Treatment of Glioma

Johnny Camargo

Abstract

Gliomas have been treated by a specialized team including neurosurgery, radiation therapy, and neuro-oncology, as well as depending on integrated sophisticated facilities and multi-professional team. Despite these huge efforts to glioma treatment, glioblastoma, one of the most frequent gliomas, has median life expectance for just 15 months, so these results are still an unmet need. Related to the systemic treatment, some cancer approaches have been revolutionized with new strategies, such as immunotherapy, although in neuro-oncology, this alternative still has challenges to overcome. Throughout this chapter, relevant information and key points will be discussed to the best way to manage systemic treatment and improve glioma overall survival.

Keywords: gliomas, glioblastoma, astrocytoma, oligodendroglioma, immunotherapy, systemic treatment, chemotherapy

1. Introduction

Gliomas are the most common primary brain tumors [1]; their origin is from glial cells, i.e., from astrocytes, oligodendrocytes, and ependymal cells. Usually, it has diffused appearance, and depending on their molecular features, they may have different behaviors. The worst evolution is related to glioblastoma, in which the best treatment might provide the dismal evolution in 15 months of overall survival (OS) [2]. On the other hand, even with diffuse infiltration, when there are astrocytic features, the OS might be up to 7 years, and with oligodendroglial features [3, 4], the OS is around more than 10 years. So, these diseases are very heterogeneous in regard to pathogenesis, histopathology, and molecular and clinical features.

Related to glioma treatment, for the optimization of results [5], it is necessary to be aware of clinical variables, such as age, sex, Karnofsky Performance Status on admission, isocitrate dehydrogenase 1/2 mutation ratio, or resection rate. Besides, there is a necessity of engaged and specialized staff of neurosurgeons, radiation therapist, neuro-oncologist, anesthetist, radiologist, and a supportive staff, in an equipped and organized structure with facilities for brain tumor care.

The systemic approaches make part of glioma treatment, using drugs with direct action in tumor cells [6, 7], in association with radiation therapy [2] aiming to potentialize it, as an adjuvant therapy [8], and currently for action in the vascular formation [9, 10] and to modulate immune system.

2. Challenges for drug efficacy in CNS tumors

The preferred treatment for brain tumors has been attempting to maximize the degree of surgical resection. But irrespective of the relevance of this approach, it

IntechOpen

has limitations with respect to gliomas due to the invasiveness of these tumors and their tendency to reside in or near important brain areas. Traditional postsurgical therapy for gliomas involved standard radiation therapy and chemotherapy. There are some issues which might be considered as a challenge to improve glioma treatment.

2.1 Blood-brain barrier (BBB), blood-cerebrospinal fluid barrier (blood-CSFB), and blood-tumor barrier

Anatomically, CNS can be subdivided into the parenchyma, meninges, special sense organs, cranial nerves, spinal nerves, and the ventricular system with its contents. All these structures are limited by boundaries under normal conditions, such as blood-brain barrier, blood-CSFB, and, in pathologic scenario, blood-tumor barrier. Under normal physiology, the BBB's unique anatomic structure and the tightly regulated interplay of its cellular and acellular components allow for maintenance of brain homeostasis, regulation of influx and efflux, and protection from harm; these characteristics ensure an optimal environment for the neural network to function properly. It is not really a barrier but rather a communication "center," responding to and passing signals between the CNS and blood [11]. It is constituted by cells that surround the vessels, the endothelium cells, which have been considered the central unit, and there is a growing understanding in the interactions of this central cell with other cells and systems, such as pericytes [12], astrocytes [13], and microglia. The integration among them results in maintenance of BBB permeability. There is a vast research to study the relation between this complex system and pathologies. Under pathologic conditions, these barriers might lose their permeability allowing easy traffic between the compartments.

Charge, lipophilicity, and molecular size are key issues for drugs to pass through BBB. Drugs currently in use for CNS tumors, for example, temozolomide and lomustine, can reach, despite BBB permeability, in areas with neoplastic enhancement in imaging studies, which might have dysfunctional BBB and permit some drugs to get in easily.

For instance, BBB is part of complex environment that supports the balance and homeostasis of CNS, and it is as well a barrier both to drugs and chemotherapeutic agents and to immunotherapeutic agents.

2.2 Drug development

The best quality preclinical testing model would select appropriate molecular targets, determine the effectiveness of drugs directed against those targets and the ideal genetic and cellular context for their use, evaluate the toxicity of selected drugs, and identify relevant biomarkers demonstrating drug efficacy and specificity to assist in subsequent clinical trials [14].

At the laboratory level, there are limitations of drug development for gliomas. Preclinical tests might be performed in in vitro tests or in animal model tests. In in vitro tests, there are limitations owing to cellular homogeneity that could not reproduce the real tumor environment and cellular heterogeneity; moreover, the systemic influences affect drug metabolism and distribution, and what's more, in an animal model in which are based on xenografts inserts in flank or directly into the animal brain. But these models, despite working in preclinical models, usually fail to reproduce the same result at the clinical level. Another strategy that has been developed by using genetically engineered mouse models (GEMMs) [15] has shown that glial tumors spontaneously develop, mostly of high grade, after a variable latent period. Such GEMMs are the best current models we have for approximating the biology of CNS neoplasms in humans.

Other efforts have been made in order to better understand the overlap of various models and human brain tumor behavior; in recent published paper [16], the authors have studied the differences and similarities in glioma biology as conveyed by transcriptomic patterns across four mammalian hosts: rats, mice, dogs, and humans. And they have found notable differences that were observed in gene expression patterns as well as related biological pathways and cell populations known to mediate key elements of glioma biology, including angiogenesis, immune evasion, and brain invasion.

2.3 Tumor heterogeneity

Tumor heterogeneity may keep tumor evolution and adaptation, which prevent personalized medicine agents to work [17]. It has been described in various tumor models, and this feature in gliomas allowed them to be resistant to several known drugs [18, 19].

There is a growing knowledge in the molecular and cellular basis of glioblastoma; Diane J. Aum [18], in her paper, introduced emerging concepts on the molecular and cellular heterogeneity of glioblastoma and laid emphasis that we should begin to consider each individual glioblastoma to be an ensemble of distinct subclones that reflect a spectrum of dynamic cell states. And this knowledge partially explains this entity's resistance to treatment, as well as allows new researches and strategies to overcome it.

2.4 Immunosuppressive environment of brain tissue

A detailed understanding of the supportive role that the microenvironment plays in glioblastoma (GBM) is critical to the design of effective immunotherapeutic strategies. Glioma histology shows that >30% of GBM tumors are composed of infiltrating microglia [20] with active recruitment of peripheral macrophages [21]. The secretion of immunomodulatory cytokines from GBM cells, including interleukins 10 (IL-10), 4 (IL-4), and 6 (IL-6), and, particularly, tumor growth factor-beta (TGF-β) in addition to prostaglandin E2 can suppress microglia activation.

Tumor-associated macrophages (TAM) [22] are often considered to be facilitators of tumor growth because of their proangiogenic and immunosuppressive properties. Besides it, the glioma tumor cells are between the least immunogenic in the spectrum of the human tumors, which confer then to be less responsive to immunotherapy [23].

Therefore, a complex system allows tumor cells to grow without immune system control, and this knowledge opens new avenues to exploration of immunotherapeutic issues.

3. Glioma classification

The new version of the World Health Organization Classification of Tumors of the Central Nervous System (WHO 2016) [24] introduced the concept of an integrated diagnosis, based on a union of both phenotypic (microscopic) and genotypic parameters. Major changes are seen in glioma and medulloblastoma groups. Fewer entities are included and some, related to their no longer diagnostic and therapeutic relevance, were deleted.

In the previous version, WHO 2007, all astrocytic tumors had been grouped together, but now in new 2016 classification, all diffuse gliomas whether they are astrocytic or oligodendroglial are grouped under one heading, mainly based on their growth pattern, behavior, as well as a mutation in IDH.

Regarding the histological classification at the WHO 2016, there were few modifications; tumors are still being classified as grade I, II, III, and IV; and just a new category "grade unknown" is added for diffuse leptomeningeal glioneuronal tumor [25].

3.1 Nomenclature

The nomenclature of the combination of histopathological and molecular features must be standardized to simplify its use; CNS tumor diagnoses should consist of a histopathological name followed by the genetic features, with the genetic features following a comma and as adjectives, as in *diffuse astrocytoma*, IDH *mutant*, and *medulloblastoma*, wingless (WNT) *activated*. If there are more than one genetic features, it must be included in the description, for example, *oligodendroglioma,* IDH *mutant* and *1p/19q co-deleted.* When the tumor has no genetic alteration, the term "wild type" might be used if an official entity already exists, for example, *glioblastoma* IDH *wild type.*

For situations which there are no access to molecular tests, or it was not done, by whatever reason, the term not otherwise specified (NOS) must be used, for example, *diffuse astrocytoma, NOS.* For instance, the NOS terminology refers to an incomplete or unavailable information related to molecular tests.

3.2 Gliomas

Despite having astrocytic or oligodendroglial features, in the WHO 2016, they are grouped together as diffuse gliomas, and for pathologic point of view, it is useful, so they are grouped together; for prognostic issues and patient management, the therapeutic orientation might be driven biologically and genetically.

Astrocytic gliomas include diffuse lesions, which may be grade II, grade III (anaplastic), and grade IV (glioblastoma), and main molecular features are IDH and alpha-thalassemia/mental retardation syndrome X-linked (ATRX) gene. IDH-mutated lesions may have better evolution. Grades II and III are mainly IDH mutated, whereas grade IV (glioblastoma) is predominately IDH wild type.

Oligodendroglial tumors have their histological features; although astrocytic ones might have its feature as well, and its molecular features are IDH mutated and 1p/19q co-deleted, these classes of tumors have better prognosis. It may have grade II and grade III (anaplastic). When the genetic tests are not available, it will be classified as diffuse astrocytoma, NOS; oligodendroglioma, NOS; or glioblastoma, NOS.

4. Glioma molecular markers

4.1 IDH1 and IDH2

IDH is the most important diagnostic marker as it can differentiate glioma from gliosis. These mutations have affected amino acid 132 of isocitrate dehydrogenase 1 gene (IDH1) in more than 70% of the WHO grade II and III astrocytomas and oligodendrogliomas and in glioblastomas that have developed from these lower-grade lesions [26].

Two IDH variants have been used, IDH1 and IDH2, which are enzymes in Krebs cycle that catalyzes the conversion of isocitrate to alpha-ketoglutarate. IDH1 mutations are heterozygous, and these are involving an amino acid substitution (glycine to arginine) in the active site of the enzyme in codon 132 (R132H). This mutation results in the abnormal production of 2-hydroxyglutarate, which causes histone and deoxyribonucleic acid (DNA) methylation, hence promoting tumorigenesis [27], while IDH2 variants are reported to influence angiogenesis, apoptosis, and glucose metabolism [28].

IDH can be demonstrated by IDH1 or IDH2 mutation by immunohistochemistry using mutation-specific antibody against R132H-mutant IDH1; if immunostaining is negative, then it should be followed by IDH1/IDH2 DNA genotyping. Mutation in both IDH1 and IDH2 entities is known as IDH mutant. When both are negative, then it is known as IDH wild type. If IDH testing is not available or cannot be fully performed or is inconclusive, then it is labeled as IDH NOS.

4.2 1p/19q co-deletion

In 1p/19q co-deletion, there is a complete deletion of both the short arm of chromosome 1 (1p) and the long arm of chromosome 19 (19q). 1p/19q co-deletion can be demonstrated by fluorescent *in situ* hybridization (FISH), polymerase chain reaction, chromogenic *in situ* hybridization, or molecular genetic testing. It is definitive for the diagnosis of grade II and grade III (anaplastic) oligodendrogliomas. It is a strong prognostic factor associated with improved survival and also a predictive factor for response to chemotherapy as well as radiotherapy [29, 30].

4.3 O6-methylguanine-DNA methyltransferase methylation (MGMT)

The MGMT gene encodes a DNA repair enzyme that can nullify the effects of alkylating chemotherapy such as temozolomide [31]. The alkylating chemotherapy damages DNA by adding methyl groups. Therefore, a tumor with a high degree of MGMT activity will be resistant to chemotherapies which target DNA at this location. If the promoter region of the MGMT gene is unmethylated, the gene will be active, whereas if the promoter region of MGMT is hypermethylated, the gene will be silenced. However, if the MGMT gene is active, the damage is rapidly repaired. Methylation of the MGMT gene promoter is a favorable prognostic and predictive factor in glioblastoma patients, but it is not a diagnostic marker for the same.

The correlation with other biomarkers is mandatory to have oriented treatment in neuro-oncology [32].

4.4 TERT (telomerase reverse transcriptase) promoter mutations

TERT mutations often involve C228T and C250T mutations of the promoter region. TERT promoter mutations and long telomere length predict poor survival and radiotherapy resistance in gliomas. It occurs mainly in glioblastoma and oligodendroglioma. TERTp and IDH mutations are routinely used clinically to facilitate diagnosis by classifying 80% of GBMs into molecular subgroups with distinct clinical courses [30, 33].

4.5 Alpha-thalassemia/mental retardation syndrome X-linked (ATRX)

It is a chromatin-remodeling protein important in DNA replication, telomere stability, gene transcription, chromosome congression, and cohesion during cell division. ATRX mutation results in lengthening of telomerase which helps in chromatin maintenance and remodeling. All cells are ATRX positive. If ATRX mutation is present, then there will be a loss of staining in the cells [34].

ATRX mutations are almost always accompanied by other mutations in the histone regulation (IDH, H33 K27M, tumor protein p53 [TP53], etc.) [35]. Loss of ATRX expression is seen in 45% of anaplastic astrocytoma, 27% of anaplastic oligoastrocytoma, and 10% of anaplastic oligodendroglioma and also in pediatric and adult high-grade astrocytoma [36].

4.6 Tumor protein p53

p53 is a tumor suppressor gene located on the short arm of chromosome 17. Loss of p53 leads to DNA damage, hypoxia, oncogene activation, microtubule disruption, and oxidative damage which in turn contributes to the CNS tumor pathogenesis mainly medulloblastoma, glioblastoma, and in 56–58% of IDH-mutant astrocytoma [37]. Copy number neutral loss of heterozygosity of chromosome 17p (CNLOH 17p) was nearly exclusively associated with IDH1-mutant astrocytoma with TP53 mutations. "CNLOH" means that one copy of the chromosome has been deleted, whereas the remaining copy has been duplicated. The net result is that the cell still has a total of two copies of the gene or chromosomal segment, but instead of having two different copies, a single copy has been duplicated. CNLOH 17p was found to be a significant prognostic factor, with better survival outcomes for those with the CNLOH 17p alteration [38].

5. Low-grade gliomas

Usually, the term "low-grade glioma" refers to the glioma class, which has an indolent evolution and an incurable disease, and during their evolution transform into a high grade. It has a specific molecular and genetic profile. In the WHO 2016, they are represented by diffuse astrocytic glioma grade II, IDH mutant and IDH wild type, and diffuse oligodendroglioma, IDH mutant with 1p/19q co-deletion or not [39].

Surgery is a key point on its management, getting tissue for biopsy and molecular analysis, and the timing depends on some variables, such as tumor size, localization, age of patient, and symptoms. Patients with small tumors might be followed regularly; despite not having randomized studies, early intervention has been showing OS advantages, as well the extension of resection and maximum safe resection rather than partial resection or biopsy [40–42].

Radiation therapy is an important part of the low-grade glioma treatment, and the optimal timing is controversial; by the way, for those ones with high risk of relapse, the immediate delivery of radiation is of the standard approaches [43].

Regarding the systemic treatment, chemotherapy is part of its treatment in the adjuvant and at relapse setting of the low-grade glioma spectrum.

In RTOG 9802, patients were randomly assigned to radiation therapy (RT) alone or RT followed by six cycles of procarbazine, lomustine, and vincristine (PCV). The primary endpoint was OS, and the secondary endpoint was PFS and grade III toxicity. At the time of the first publication [44] with a median follow-up of 5.9 years in surviving patients, there was a trend toward longer survival in the RT plus chemotherapy group (5-year overall survival 72 vs. 63%, hazard ratio [HR] 0.72, 95% CI 0.47–1.10), but with a median follow-up of 11.9 years showed at second publication [45], the significance of OS and progression-free survival (PFS) was reached, with median overall survival 13.3 vs. 7.8 years for patients treated with RT followed by

PCV, HR 0.59, p = 0.03, and the median progression-free survival was also prolonged in patients who received PCV (10.4 vs. 4.0 years, p = 0.002).

These results bring level 1 evidence to treat high-risk patients with low-grade gliomas with RT and PCV. As PCV is toxic and there are further evidences of equivalences with temozolomide [46], despite not being randomized by studies comparing it in this population, this drug can be used with the 2B level of evidence. At CATNON trial, there was a comparison in patients with anaplastic oligodendrogliomas with no co-deletion, between RT and RT followed by temozolomide, with OS advantage.

In the subgroup of patients who had had 1p/19q co-deletion, the significance of benefit from PCV was greater in patients with oligodendroglioma (n = 101; HR 0.43, 95% CI 0.23–0.82) and oligoastrocytoma (n = 77; HR 0.56, 95% CI 0.32–1.0) than in those with astrocytoma (n = 46; HR 0.73, 95% CI 0.40–1.34).

6. High-grade gliomas

This category is composed by grade III diffuse gliomas (anaplastic astrocytoma, anaplastic oligodendroglioma) and grade IV (glioblastoma). Typically, the symptom evolution occurs in few weeks or months. Among them, there are different prognoses, so as anaplastic oligodendroglioma has OS of 9 years, anaplastic astrocytoma has OS of 3–5 years, and glioblastoma has OS of just 15 months. The prognosis will be dependent on age, performance status, localization of the lesion, grade of resection [47, 48], and molecular profile for grade III diffuse gliomas (IDH and 1p/19q co-deletion) and for glioblastoma (IDH status, MGMT, TERT, p53, epidermal growth factor receptor variant III (EGFRvIII), and others).

Surgery for high-grade gliomas has the goal of maximum safe resection [49], with prognosis improvement, or at least partial resection or stereotactic biopsy to define histology, as well as molecular markers to drive treatment. Many strategies have been tested to reach maximum safe resection, such as awake surgery, intraoperative magnetic resonance [50], 5-aminolevulinic acid (5-ALA) guide surgery [48], and other techniques that require expertise and facilities to deal with these demands.

Further adjuvant treatment, considering gold standard, using radiation therapy and systemic treatment is required. To revisit this issue, it might be considered that previous trials took data from a mix of histologic and molecular subtypes, not taking in account the updated WHO 2016.

6.1 Grade III diffuse gliomas

6.1.1 Anaplastic oligodendroglioma

In this subtype, the knowledge of the role of 1p/19q co-deletion as better prognostic marker as far has been demonstrated [51]. According to the WHO 2016, this tumor must have IDH mutation and 1p/19q co-deletion.

One of the evidences to treat this class of patient with combination of radiation therapy and chemotherapy was demonstrated in EORTC brain tumor group study 26951 [29], where 368 adult patients with newly diagnosed anaplastic oligodendroglial tumors were randomly assigned to either RT or the same RT followed by six cycles of adjuvant PCV, and with a median follow-up of 140 months, OS in the RT/PCV arm was significantly longer (42.3 vs. 30.6 months in the RT arm, hazard ratio [HR], 0.75; 95% CI, 0.60–0.95). In an exploratory analysis of 80 patients with a 1p/19q co-deletion, OS was increased, with a trend toward more benefits from adjuvant PCV (OS not reached in the RT/PCV group vs. 112 months in the RT group; HR, 0.56; 95% CI, 0.31–1.03). IDH mutational status was also of prognostic significance.

At RTOG 9402 in an updated publication [52], 291 patients with anaplastic oligodendrogliomas and pure (AO) and mixed (anaplastic oligoastrocytoma (AOA) were randomized to four cycles of PCV followed by radiation therapy (RT). For the entire cohort, there was no difference in median survival by treatment (4.6 years for PCV plus RT vs. 4.7 years for RT), but for 1p/19q co-deleted patients as in EORTC 26951, there was survival benefit, although this analysis was not preplanned.

6.1.2 Anaplastic astrocytoma

In the WHO 2016, anaplastic astrocytoma molecular feature is IDH1/IDH2 mutated and IDH1/IDH2 wild type, with no 1p/19q co-deletion. Anaplastic astrocytoma IDH1/IDH2 wild type has worse prognosis than the IDH1/IDH-2 mutated [25].

At CATNON trial (EORTC study 26053-22054) [8], 745 patients (99%) of the planned 748 patients, with anaplastic astrocytoma with no 1p/19q co-deletion, had been enrolled in a four-arm study comparing RT alone, RT with concurrent daily temozolomide, RT followed by 12 cycles of adjuvant temozolomide, and RT with both concurrent and 12 cycles of adjuvant temozolomide. At the interim analysis of RT × RT followed by 12 cycles of adjuvant temozolomide, the temozolomide addition had a significant improvement in both progression-free survival (HR 0.62, 95% CI 0.50–0.76) and overall survival (median 44.1 months vs. not yet reached; HR 0.65, 95% CI 0.45–0.93).

So, based upon CATNON trial and other observations [53, 54], patients with anaplastic astrocytoma must be treated with adjuvant RT and chemotherapy, and if IDH is wild type, it must be treated as glioblastoma. To IDH-mutated lesions, until final analysis of CATNON trial, there is no evidence-based data supporting concomitant adjuvant treatment for this subgroup.

6.2 Grade IV gliomas: glioblastoma

Glioblastoma has been a daily challenge for those who attend these patients, as well for those who are involved in research area. Glioblastoma is the most common glioma and usually has dismal evolution in few months or years, so it has OS of just 15 months. At the Stupp trial [2], in the current standard of care of postoperative therapy for glioblastoma, 573 newly diagnosed patients with histologically confirmed glioblastoma were randomly assigned to receive radiotherapy alone or radiotherapy plus continuous daily temozolomide, followed by six cycles of adjuvant temozolomide. At a median follow-up of 28 months, the median survival was 14.6 months with radiotherapy plus temozolomide and 12.1 months with radiotherapy alone. The unadjusted hazard ratio for death in the radiotherapy plus temozolomide group was 0.63 (95% confidence interval, 0.52–0.75; $P < 0.001$ by the log-rank test).

At this trial and others [55, 56], MGMT-methylated patients are doing better, and this biomarker became a strong predictor of temozolomide response.

Low-intensity alternating electric field therapy (TTFields) is a novel treatment to glioblastoma, in which locoregionally delivered antimitotic treatment interferes with cell division and organelle assembly. This stimulus is delivered continuously by transducers applied to a shaved scalp. In an open-label randomized trial of 695 adults with newly diagnosed glioblastoma, median survival was improved in patients assigned to wear the device during the adjuvant temozolomide phase of standard chemoradiation compared with those assigned to standard chemoradiation alone (21 vs. 16 months) [57, 58]. The requirement to carry a device and maintain a shaved scalp for the duration of treatment presents a potential burden that is not acceptable to all patients [59].

On a phase II study [60], 39 glioblastoma patients are offered with radiotherapy of tumor site only and CCNU/TMZ (carmustine/temozolomide) chemotherapy for up to six courses. It results in a longer survival when compared to historical controls, mainly in MGMT-methylated patients; in the whole cohort, the median overall survival (mOS) was 23.1 months, and comparing MGMT methylated or not, the mOS was significantly longer with 34.3 vs. 12.5 months. The WHO grade IV hematologic toxicity was frequent.

CeTeG/NOA-09 trial was designed to prove that MGMT-methylated glioblastoma patients might have better survival using CCNU/TMZ. In this trial, there was randomization between MGMT-methylated glioblastoma patients to treat with a standard Stupp protocol vs. six cycles of CCNU/TMZ, its results were presented at plenary section of 22nd SNO (Society of Neuro-oncology meeting) [61], and it results in mOS for TMZ of 30.4 and 46.9 months for CCNU/TMZ. These are challenging results, waiting for publication for further details.

7. New strategies to treat gliomas

In the last 30 years, there have been huge investments in glioma research for better outcomes; despite being fruitful, it is far from being solved. There are studies in anti-angiogenic drugs, inhibition of integrins, inhibition of growth factor receptors and intracellular signaling pathways, and immunotherapy, and despite failing to improve OS, immunotherapy has demonstrated hopeful results.

Immunotherapy has been extensively studied, with better understanding of relationship between tumors and immune system [62], and it is totally clear that immune system plays a key role in the tumor evolution as well as its control. Currently, immunotherapy has been standard in a growing spectrum of tumors [63, 64].

Immunotherapy challenges in glioblastoma, owing to low mutational load (TML) and therefore potential immunogenicity, and tight immune regulation within the CNS result in limited T-cell effector responses, which means that immunosuppressive microenvironment and blockade of some cells to CNS have been limited for better use of this strategy in glioma field.

7.1 Vaccines

As an active immunotherapy (vaccine), rindopepimut (Rintega) consists of an EGFRvIII peptide conjugated to keyhole limpet hemocyanin, which is expressed in 30% of cells from glioblastoma patients and was previously tested in a phase II trial (ACT III) [65], and it had been the first immunotherapeutic to demonstrate increased survival. The hypothesis had been tested in a phase III trial, ACT IV [66], in which patients with newly diagnosed GBM with EGFRvIII expressed treated with standard chemoradiation with or without rindopepimut. Its publication showed that there was no difference at primary endpoint, with OS of 20.4 vs. 21.1 months. There are some evidences of association between bevacizumab and rindopepimut having synergistic effect [67], but this hypothesis must be proven.

Another provocative strategy has just been published [68] in a phase III trial which evaluates the addition of an autologous tumor lysate-pulsed dendritic cell vaccine (DCVax®-L) to standard therapy for newly diagnosed glioblastoma.

The final results are not yet available, because they are still unblinded, until the sufficient events have occurred to elucidate the final curves. Despite being an interim analysis, it has been shown 23.4 months of medium OS (mOS), as the intention-to-treat (ITT) population is similar, and it was allowed to crossover. So, we have to wait for the final data.

7.2 Checkpoint inhibitors

Another promising area is immunotherapy with checkpoint inhibitors, although a recent trial failed to demonstrate survival benefit. The CheckMate 143 was the first randomized phase III clinical trial in GBM with a PD-1 checkpoint inhibitor. In nivolumab alone vs. bevacizumab alone in recurrent GBM, 369 patients were randomized to the nivolumab (n = 184) or bevacizumab (n = 185), resulting in a median OS of 9.8 months with nivolumab and 10 months with bevacizumab, and the 12-month OS rate was 42% in both arms. Despite having failed to demonstrate advantage, in a specific scenario, in patients with biallelic mismatch repair deficiency (bMMRD), it can benefit from checkpoint inhibitor treatment [69]. This might be explained by a high mutational burden in bMMRD. In other considerations, CheckMate 143 failure involves an inability of nivolumab to reach tumor-infiltrating lymphocytes (TILs) already sequestered in the recurrent tumor microenvironment; it may be expected to function better in patients with newly diagnosed GBM, where newly activated circulating T cells would be available for interaction with nivolumab prior to their migration to tumor sites. So, further investigation is required to set PD-1 checkpoint in glioma treatment [70, 71].

7.3 CAR T cells

Tumor immunotherapy with T lymphocytes, which can recognize and destroy malignant cells, has been limited by the ability to isolate and expand T cells restricted to tumor-associated antigens. Chimeric antigen receptors (CARs) composed of antibody-binding domains connected to domains that activate T cells could overcome tolerance by allowing T cells to respond to cell surface antigens; however, to date, lymphocytes engineered to express CARs have demonstrated minimal in vivo expansion and antitumor effects in clinical trials [72]. The very begging publications related to CAR T-cell therapy were related to a relapsed and refractory acute lymphoblastic leukemia, which made this technology known.

At glioma setting, CAR T-cell therapy has been tested, in recurrent GBM utilizing CAR T-cell GBM-associated antigen IL13Ra2 that utilizes CD62L-enriched central memory T cells (Tcm) engineered by lentiviral transduction to express [73]. Second-generation 4-1BB-containing CAR (IL13BBZ) signaling domain was utilized by both intratumoral and intraventricular deliveries, with multiple doses via reservoir. Safely and well tolerated, some dramatic responses were observed, both in brain and meninx lesions.

Further efforts have been made to improve results of this therapy [74–76].

7.4 Cancer-targeting oncolytic viruses

Cancer virotherapy mediated by oncolytic viruses (OV) has emerged as a novel and effective strategy in cancer therapeutics [77]. Desjardins [78] in a dose-finding and toxicity phase I study evaluated an intratumoral delivery of the recombinant nonpathogenic poliovirus-rhinovirus chimera (PVSRIPO). PVSRIPO recognizes the poliovirus receptor CD155, which is widely expressed in neoplastic cells of solid tumors and in major components of the tumor microenvironment. Overall survival among the patients who received PVSRIPO reached a plateau of 21% (95% confidence interval, 11–33) at 24 months that was sustained at 36 months. For glioma grade IV with standard treatment, there is no plateau. A phase II study in this setting is ongoing NCT02986178.

8. Conclusions

Glioma treatment is still a challenge, and its quality is related to integrated team, in which the systemic treatment must be based on awareness of drug limitation usage and keeping in mind strategies to overcome these issues.

Conflict of interest

The author declares no conflict of interests.

Notes/thanks/other declarations

Thanks for those colleagues who based on their professionalism, dedication, future vision, engagement, and commitment have been an example to be followed and have made this task easier, as well as to brain tumor patients and their families, for whom all the efforts are being made.

Author details

Johnny Camargo[1,2]*

1 Curitiba's Neurologic Institute (INC), Parana's Oncology Institute (IOP), Curitiba, Brazil

2 Brazilian Society of Clinical Oncology, American Society of Clinical Oncology, Brazil

*Address all correspondence to: jfccamargo@gmail.com

IntechOpen

© 2018 The Author(s). Licensee IntechOpen. This chapter is distributed under the terms of the Creative Commons Attribution License (http://creativecommons.org/licenses/by/3.0), which permits unrestricted use, distribution, and reproduction in any medium, provided the original work is properly cited. CC BY

References

[1] Ostrom QT et al. CBTRUS statistical report: Primary brain and central nervous system tumors diagnosed in the United States in 2007-2011. Neuro-Oncology. 2014;**16**(Suppl 4):iv1-i63

[2] Stupp R et al. Radiotherapy plus concomitant and adjuvant temozolomide for glioblastoma. The New England Journal of Medicine. 2005;**352**(10):987-996

[3] Olson JD, Riedel E, DeAngelis LM. Long-term outcome of low-grade oligodendroglioma and mixed glioma. Neurology. 2000;**54**(7):1442-1448

[4] Bauman G et al. Adult supratentorial low-grade glioma: Long-term experience at a single institution. International Journal of Radiation Oncology, Biology, Physics. 2009;**75**(5):1401-1407

[5] Pollom EL et al. Newly diagnosed glioblastoma: Adverse socioeconomic factors correlate with delay in radiotherapy initiation and worse overall survival. Journal of Radiation Research. 2018;**59**(suppl_1):i11-i18

[6] Yung WK. Temozolomide in malignant gliomas. Seminars in Oncology. 2000;**27**(3 Suppl 6):27-34

[7] Friedman HS, Kerby T, Calvert H. Temozolomide and treatment of malignant glioma. Clinical Cancer Research. 2000;**6**(7):2585-2597

[8] van den Bent MJ et al. Interim results from the CATNON trial (EORTC study 26053-22054) of treatment with concurrent and adjuvant temozolomide for 1p/19q non-co-deleted anaplastic glioma: A phase 3, randomised, open-label intergroup study. The Lancet. 2017;**390**(10103):1645-1653

[9] Liu Y et al. Improvement of health related quality of life in patients with recurrent glioma treated with bevacizumab plus daily temozolomide as the salvage therapy. Clinical Neurology and Neurosurgery. 2018;**169**:64-70

[10] Winkler F, Osswald M, Wick W. Anti-angiogenics: Their role in the treatment of glioblastoma. Oncology Research and Treatment. 2018;**41**(4):181-186

[11] Keaney J, Campbell M. The dynamic blood-brain barrier. The FEBS Journal. 2015;**282**(21):4067-4079

[12] Nakagawa S et al. Pericytes from brain microvessels strengthen the barrier integrity in primary cultures of rat brain endothelial cells. Cellular and Molecular Neurobiology. 2007;**27**:687-694

[13] Placone AL et al. Human astrocytes develop physiological morphology and remain quiescent in a novel 3D matrix. Biomaterials. 2015;**42**:134-143

[14] Sharpless NE, Depinho RA. The mighty mouse: Genetically engineered mouse models in cancer drug development. Nature Reviews. Drug Discovery. 2006;**5**(9):741-754

[15] Huse JT, Holland EC. Genetically engineered mouse models of brain cancer and the promise of preclinical testing. Brain Pathology (Zurich, Switzerland). 2009;**19**(1):132-143

[16] Connolly NP et al. Cross-species transcriptional analysis reveals conserved and host-specific neoplastic processes in mammalian glioma. Scientific Reports. 2018;**8**:1180

[17] Gerlinger M et al. Intratumor heterogeneity and branched evolution revealed by multiregion sequencing. New England Journal of Medicine. 2012;**366**(10):883-892

[18] Aum DJ et al. Molecular and cellular heterogeneity: The hallmark of glioblastoma. Neurosurgical Focus. 2014;**37**(6):E11

[19] Patel AP et al. Single-cell RNA-seq highlights intratumoral heterogeneity in primary glioblastoma. Science. 2014;**344**(6190):1396-1401

[20] Watters JJ, Schartner JM, Behnam B. Microglia function in brain tumors. Journal of Neuroscience Research. 2005;**81**(3):447-455

[21] Atai AN et al. Osteopontin is up-regulated and associated with neutrophil and macrophage infiltration in glioblastoma. Immunology. 2011;**132**(1):39-48

[22] Chen Z, Hambardzumyan D. Immune microenvironment in glioblastoma subtypes. Frontiers in Immunology. 2018;**9**:1004

[23] Reardon DA, Wen PY. Unravelling tumour heterogeneity—Implications for therapy. Nature Reviews. Clinical Oncology. 2015;**12**:69

[24] Louis DN et al. The 2016 world health organization classification of tumors of the central nervous system: A summary. Acta Neuropathologica. 2016;**131**(6):803-820

[25] Komori T. The 2016 WHO classification of tumours of the central nervous system: The major points of revision. Neurologia Medico-Chirurgica (Tokyo). 2017;**57**(7):301-311

[26] Hai Yan D et al. IDH1 and IDH2 mutations in gliomas. The New England Journal of Medicine. 2009;**360**:765-773

[27] Guo C et al. Isocitrate dehydrogenase mutations in gliomas: Mechanisms, biomarkers and therapeutic target. Current Opinion in Neurology. 2011;**24**(6):648-652

[28] van Thuijl HF et al. Genetics and pharmacogenomics of diffuse gliomas. Pharmacology & Therapeutics. 2013;**137**(1):78-88

[29] van den Bent MJ et al. Adjuvant procarbazine, lomustine, and vincristine chemotherapy in newly diagnosed anaplastic oligodendroglioma: Long-term follow-up of EORTC brain tumor group study 26951. Journal of Clinical Oncology. 2013;**31**(3):344-350

[30] Eckel-Passow JE et al. Glioma groups based on 1p/19q, IDH, and TERT promoter mutations in tumors. The New England Journal of Medicine. 2015;**372**(26):2499-2508

[31] Cankovic M et al. The role of *MGMT* testing in clinical practice. The Journal of Molecular Diagnostics. 2013;**15**(5):539-555

[32] Wick W et al. Prognostic or predictive value of *MGMT* promoter methylation in gliomas depends on *IDH1* mutation. Neurology. 2013;**81**(17):1515-1522

[33] Killela PJ et al. Mutations in IDH1, IDH2, and in the TERT promoter define clinically distinct subgroups of adult malignant gliomas. Öncotarget. 2014;**5**(6):1515-1565

[34] The Cancer Genome Atlas Research, N. Comprehensive, integrative genomic analysis of diffuse lower-grade gliomas. The New England Journal of Medicine. 2015;**372**(26):2481-2498

[35] Diplas BH et al. The genomic landscape of TERT promoter wildtype-IDH wildtype glioblastoma. Nature Communications. 2018;**9**(1):2087

[36] Haase S et al. Mutant ATRX: Uncovering a new therapeutic target for glioma. Expert Opinion on Therapeutic Targets. 2018;**22**(7):599-613

[37] Kondo T. Molecular mechanisms involved in gliomagenesis. Brain Tumor Pathology. 2017;**34**(1):1-7

[38] Lin T et al. The expression of p53, mgmt and egfr in brain glioma and clinical significance. Journal of Biological Regulators and Homeostatic Agents. 2015;**29**(1):143-149

[39] Louis DN et al. WHO Classification of Tumours of the Central Nervous System. 4th ed. Lyon: IARC; 2016

[40] Aghi MK et al. The role of surgery in the management of patients with diffuse low grade glioma: A systematic review and evidence-based clinical practice guideline. Journal of Neuro-Oncology. 2015;**125**(3):503-530

[41] McGirt MJ et al. Extent of surgical resection is independently associated with survival in patients with hemispheric infiltrating low-grade gliomas. Neurosurgery. 2008;**63**(4):700-707; author reply 707-8

[42] Zetterling M et al. Prognostic markers for survival in patients with oligodendroglial tumors; a single-institution review of 214 cases. PLoS One. 2017;**12**(11):e0188419

[43] Ryken TC et al. The role of radiotherapy in the management of patients with diffuse low grade glioma: A systematic review and evidence-based clinical practice guideline. Journal of Neuro-Oncology. 2015;**125**(3):551-583

[44] Shaw EG et al. Randomized trial of radiation therapy plus procarbazine, lomustine, and vincristine chemotherapy for supratentorial adult low-grade glioma: Initial results of RTOG 9802. Journal of Clinical Oncology. 2012;**30**(25):3065-3070

[45] Buckner JC et al. Radiation plus procarbazine, CCNU, and vincristine in low-grade glioma. The New England Journal of Medicine. 2016;**374**(14):1344-1355

[46] Fisher BJ et al. Phase 2 study of temozolomide-based chemoradiation therapy for high-risk low-grade gliomas: Preliminary results of radiation therapy oncology group 0424. International Journal of Radiation Oncology, Biology, Physics. 2015;**91**(3):497-504

[47] Brown TJ et al. Association of the extent of resection with survival in glioblastoma: A systematic review and meta-analysis. JAMA Oncology. 2016;**2**(11):1460-1469

[48] Stummer W et al. Fluorescence-guided surgery with 5-aminolevulinic acid for resection of malignant glioma: A randomised controlled multicentre phase III trial. The Lancet Oncology. 2006;**7**(5):392-401

[49] Trifiletti DM et al. Prognostic implications of extent of resection in glioblastoma: Analysis from a large database. World Neurosurgery. 2017;**103**:330-340

[50] Ramina R et al. Optimizing costs of intraoperative magnetic resonance imaging. A series of 29 glioma cases. Acta Neurochirurgica. 2010;**152**(1):27-33

[51] Dubbink HJ et al. Molecular classification of anaplastic oligodendroglioma using next-generation sequencing: A report of the prospective randomized EORTC brain tumor group 26951 phase III trial. Neuro-Oncology. 2016;**18**(3):388-400

[52] Cairncross G et al. Phase III trial of chemoradiotherapy for anaplastic oligodendroglioma: Long-term results of RTOG 9402. Journal of Clinical Oncology. 2013;**31**(3):337-343

[53] Shin JY, Diaz AZ. Anaplastic astrocytoma: Prognostic factors and survival in 4807 patients with emphasis

on receipt and impact of adjuvant therapy. Journal of Neuro-Oncology. 2016;**129**(3):557-565

[54] Juratli TA et al. Radio-chemotherapy improves survival in IDH-mutant, 1p/19q non-codeleted secondary high-grade astrocytoma patients. Journal of Neuro-Oncology. 2015;**124**(2):197-205

[55] Stupp R et al. Effects of radiotherapy with concomitant and adjuvant temozolomide versus radiotherapy alone on survival in glioblastoma in a randomised phase III study: 5-year analysis of the EORTC-NCIC trial. The Lancet Oncology. 2009;**10**(5):459-466

[56] Hart MG et al. Temozolomide for high grade glioma. Cochrane Database of Systematic Reviews. 2013;(4):Cd007415

[57] Stupp R et al. Maintenance therapy with tumor-treating fields plus temozolomide vs. temozolomide alone for glioblastoma: A randomized clinical trial. JAMA. 2015;**314**(23):2535-2543

[58] Magouliotis DE et al. Tumor-treating fields as a fourth treating modality for glioblastoma: A meta-analysis. Acta Neurochirurgica. 2018;**160**(6):1167-1174

[59] Onken J et al. Acceptance and compliance of TTFields treatment among high grade glioma patients. Journal of Neuro-Oncology. 2018;**139**(1):177-184

[60] Glas M et al. Long-term survival of patients with glioblastoma treated with radiotherapy and lomustine plus temozolomide. Journal of Clinical Oncology. 2009;**27**(8):1257-1261

[61] Herrlinger U et al. Phase III trial of CCNU/temozolomide (TMZ) combination therapy vs. standard TMZ therapy for newly diagnosed MGMT-methylated glioblastoma patients: The CeTeg/NOA-09 trial. Neuro-Oncology. 2017;**19**(suppl_6):vi13-vi14

[62] Escors D. Tumour immunogenicity, antigen presentation and immunological barriers in cancer immunotherapy. New Journal of Science. 2014;**2014**:1-25

[63] Drake CG, Lipson EJ, Brahmer JR. Breathing new life into immunotherapy: Review of melanoma, lung and kidney cancer. Nature Reviews. Clinical Oncology. 2013;**11**(1):24-37

[64] Robert C et al. Nivolumab in previously untreated melanoma without BRAF mutation.pdf. New England Journal of Medicine. 2016;**372**(4):320-330

[65] Zussman BM, Engh JA. Outcomes of the ACT III study: Rindopepimut (CDX-110) therapy for glioblastoma. Neurosurgery. 2015;**76**(6):N17

[66] Weller M et al. Rindopepimut with temozolomide for patients with newly diagnosed, EGFRvIII-expressing glioblastoma (ACT IV): A randomised, double-blind, international phase 3 trial. The Lancet Oncology. 2017;**18**(10):1373-1385

[67] Gatson NT, Weathers SP, de Groot JF. ReACT phase II trial: A critical evaluation of the use of rindopepimut plus bevacizumab to treat EGFRvIII-positive recurrent glioblastoma. CNS Oncology. 2016;**5**(1):11-26

[68] Emerich DF, Rl D, Osborn C, Bartus RT. The development of the bradykinin agonist labradimil as a means to increase the permeability of the blood-brain barrier: From concept to clinical evaluation. Clinical Pharmacokinetics. 2001;**40**(2):105-123

[69] Bouffet E et al. Immune checkpoint inhibition for hypermutant glioblastoma multiforme resulting from germline biallelic mismatch repair deficiency. Journal of Clinical Oncology. 2016;**34**(19):2206-2211

[70] Filley AC, Henriquez M, Dey M. Recurrent glioma clinical trial, CheckMate-143: The game is not over yet. Oncotarget. 2017;**8**(53):91779-91794

[71] Mirzaei R, Sarkar S, Yong VW. T cell exhaustion in glioblastoma: Intricacies of immune checkpoints. Trends in Immunology. 2017;**38**(2):104-115

[72] Maude SL et al. Chimeric antigen receptor T cells for sustained remissions in leukemia. The New England Journal of Medicine. 2014;**371**(16):1507-1517

[73] Brown CE et al. Regression of glioblastoma after chimeric antigen receptor T-cell therapy. The New England Journal of Medicine. 2016;**375**(26):2561-2569

[74] Harris M et al. Emerging patents in the therapeutic areas of glioma and glioblastoma. Expert Opinion on Therapeutic Patents. 2018;**28**(7):573-590

[75] Sahin A et al. Development of third generation anti-EGFRvIII chimeric T cells and EGFRvIII-expressing artificial antigen presenting cells for adoptive cell therapy for glioma. PLoS One. 2018;**13**(7):e0199414

[76] Wang D et al. Glioblastoma-targeted CD4+ CAR T cells mediate superior antitumor activity. JCI Insight. 2018;**3**(10)

[77] Lin CZ et al. Advances in the mechanisms of action of cancer-targeting oncolytic viruses. Oncology Letters. 2018;**15**(4):4053-4060

[78] Desjardins A et al. Recurrent glioblastoma treated with recombinant poliovirus. The New England Journal of Medicine. 2018;**379**:150-161

Chapter 8

Role of Radiotherapy in High Grade Glioma

Henrique Balloni

Abstract

The aim of this review is to explore the changing utility of radiotherapy in the treatment of patients with glioblastoma over the past decades. Surgery and radiotherapy has always been the cornerstone of treatment of glioblastoma, but techniques have significantly advanced over this time. We selected the main studies that support the advances of radiotherapy in the present day as well as controversies in several aspects of the treatment will be approached; definition of the target volume in the magnetic resonance imaging (MRI) planning, size of the margins around the target volume; prescribed dose (satnadard vs. hypofactionated); management of glioblastoma in elderly; review role of radiosurgery past and new potential use in recurrence and the evidence of reirradiation in patients with local recurrence. Finally, continued development on many fronts have allowed for modestly improved outcomes while at the same time limiting toxicity.

Keywords: glioblastoma, radiotherapy, target volume, hypofractionated, radiosurgery

1. Introduction

The benefit of radiation therapy in patients with newly diagnosed glioblastoma has been demonstrated in many randomized trials and has been the basis of treatment for decades. To make an effort to achieve and improve the very poor outcomes associated with this disease, numerous therapeutics have been added to radiation though with lack of success until the landmark study by Stupp et al. [1] established a standard of care of treatment, gross surgical excision followed by concurrent temozolomide and radiation.

The use of radiation in glioblastoma is constantly evolving as a result of advances in imaging methods and personalized medicine leading to continuous controversies over the delineations of tumor volume.

Multiple recent studies on personalized medicine, especially in elderly patients with glioblastoma suggest that the role and dose/fractionation of radiation delivery to this increasing population will continue to develop. This chapter will highlight the major historical studies that have resulted in radiation being the current standard of care; discuss the continuing controversies of volume delineation in radiation delivery planning; discuss dose evolution and fractionation of radiotherapy in the management of patients; and review studies and ongoing trials on the use of radiation in the salvage scenario.

2. Radiotherapy target volume definitions

In the 1970s, a randomized trial showed that 60 Gy of postoperative whole-brain RT (WBRT) could improve the survival for patients with high-grade glioma (HGG). Since then, postoperative RT was a standard treatment for newly diagnosed HGG. [2] However, other studies started to compare WBRT with partial-brain irradiation and concluded that there was no advantage of WBRT [3]. Tomography (CT) and magnetic resonance imaging (MRI) has contributed largely to improve the accuracy of tumor delineation and establish that partial-brain irradiation standard to treat HGG [4]. The three-dimensional (3D) conformal radiation technique makes partial-brain irradiation for glioma possible and reduces neurotoxicity [5]. The image fusion pre- and postoperative MRI with planning CT images is normally used to determine the RT treatment volume for GBM. However, the optimal treatment volume for GBM remains a controversial issue and varies among different institutions. The Radiation Therapy Oncology Group (RTOG) refers to a two-phase treatment at 60 Gy, where the initial clinical target volume (CTV) typically includes postoperative peritumoral edema plus a 2 cm margin, followed by a boost field defined as the residual tumor plus a 2 cm margin (as per RTOG 0525 and RTOG 0825 trials) [6]. Inversely, the European Organization for Research and Treatment of Cancer (EORTC) defines a single-phase treatment with 2–3 cm dosimetric margins around the tumor (as evaluated by MRI), because 80–90% of treatment failures occur within this margin [1]. The University of Texas MD Anderson Cancer Center uses a 2 cm margin around the gross tumor volume (GTV), which consists of the resection cavity and any residual contrast-enhancing tumor without regard to edema [7]. However, several studies have raised the hypothesis that the results are similar when using reduced margins as small as 5 mm to delineate the CTV in the treatment of GBM [8].

In daily clinical practice between different institutions, the margins of the planned target volume vary significantly. A survey of radiation oncologists in Canada showed that 32 and 14% followed the RTOG and EORTC guidelines, respectively, while 54% followed the center's specific guidelines. Biphasic treatments were reported by 37% and single-phase by 60% of clinicians. For clinicians treating in single phase, 61% treat the surgical cavity and enhancing tumor with a margin, and 33% treat an area that includes tumor edema in addition to the surgical cavity and enhancing tumor. The GTV margins to generate the planning treatment volume (PTV) also varied widely and included 0.5 cm (6%), 1 cm (6%), 1.5 cm (25%), 2 cm (56%), 2.5 cm (25%), and 3 cm (12.5%). For clinicians treating in multiple phases, 90% include peritumoral edema in Phase I of the treatment. In Phase II, respondents reported using total margins (from GTV to PTV) of 1 cm (10%), 2 cm (40%), 2.5 cm (30%), and 3 cm (20%) [9]. Examples of differences in guidelines are shown (**Table 1** and **Figures 1** and **2**).

2.1 Peritumoral edema

It is discussed regarding the inclusion of edema in the treatment plan. The rationale for including peritumoral edema is that such areas are believed to contain high concentrations of tumor cells. A study compared the histopathologic distributions of neoplastic cells in GBM with the corresponding CT images and found that the vast majority of the neoplastic tissue was contained within the contrast-enhancing and low-density peritumoral areas; however, the CT low-density area was not always identical to the area infiltrated by tumor cells. No tumor cells were found in some areas of low density, whereas, in some instances, normal appearing brain tissue beyond the CT low-density area was also found to contain tumor cells [10]. Furthermore, Halperin et al. [11] compared preoperative CT scans with the postmortem topography of recurrent tumors and found that 9/11 (81.8%) tumor cells were found beyond the enhancement area plus a 1 cm margin on CT. Indeed,

Clinical Trial	CTV Margin	RT Dose
RTOG(9)	T2+ 2cm (pink) T1+2.5 cm (Red)	46 Gy 14 Gy
EORTC(4)	T1+2-3 cm (Green)	60 Gy
MD Anderson(10)	T1+ 2 cm (yellow)	60 Gy
Atlanta(11)	T2+0,7 cm T1+0,5 cm (blue)	46Gy or 54Gy 60 Gy

Table 1.
The definition of radiation treatment volumes during the delineation of high-grade gliomas.

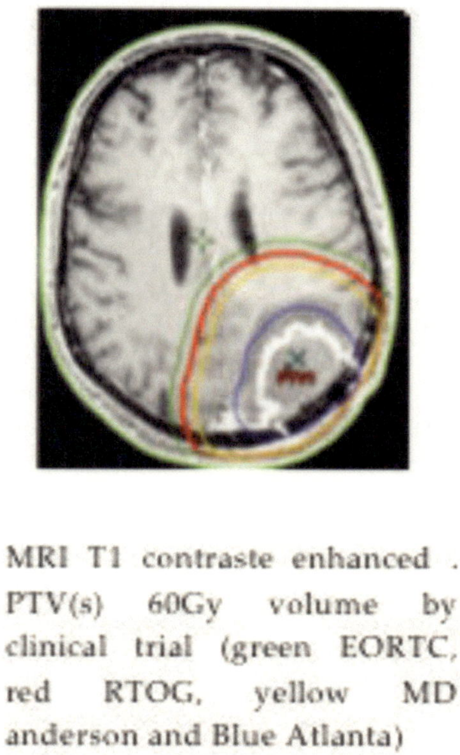

Figure 1.
Example planning treatment volumes (PTV) delineation of high grade. MRI T1 contrast enhanced showing in colors lines different protocol volumes.

only treatment plans that covered the contrast-enhancing tumor, the "edema" volume, plus an additional 3 cm margin would cover the entire histologically identified tumor. Kelly et al. [12] also reported on the correlation between histopathologic and MRI findings for 177 biopsy specimens from 39 patients with glial neoplasms. Pathologic evaluation of biopsy specimens obtained from various locations in the volumes defined by CT and MRI showed that contrast enhancement most

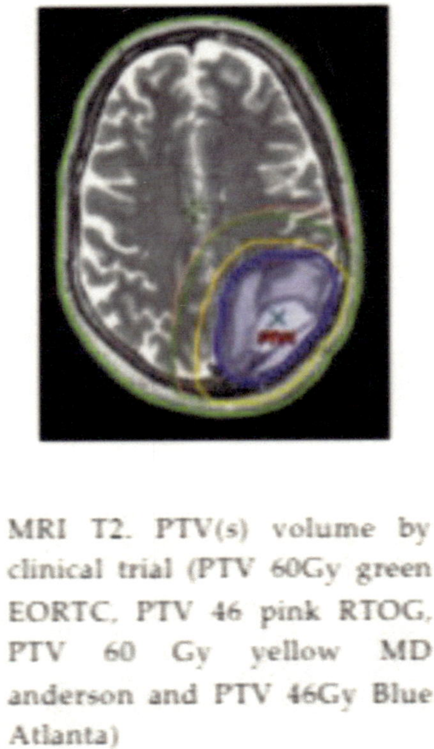

Figure 2.
Example planning treatment volumes (PTV) delineation of high grade. MRI T2 showing in colors lines different protocols volumes

often corresponded to tumor tissue without intervening parenchyma, whereas hypodensity corresponded to parenchyma infiltrated by isolated tumor cells or, in some instances, in low-HGGs, to tumor tissue or to edema. For the normal T1- and T2-weighted MRI regions that were biopsied, there was a false-negative rate of 69 and 40%, respectively [13]. A study conducted by Lu et al. [13] analyzed peritumoral edema using diffusion tensor MR imaging. This group divided gliomas associated with peritumoral edema into tumor-infiltrated edema and purely vasogenic edema.

It is controversial the prognostic of peritumoral edema. Some authors considered peritumoral edema on a preoperative MRI to be an independent prognostic factor, in addition to the postoperative Karnofsky performance score (KPS), age, and type of tumor resection [14]. Patients with major edema (>1 cm) had a significant shorter overall survival (OS) time, compared to patients with minor edema (<1 cm). Another study established that peritumoral edema, noncontrast-enhancing tumor, satellites, and multifocality were independent prognostic factors for survival in GBM, whereas preoperative tumor size, tumor location, and extent of necrosis had no significant impact on survival [15]. Conversely, there was no correlation between peritumoral edema, patient age, and tumor volume, but there was an association between edema, tumor location, and necrosis [16]. Similarly, Ramakrishna et al. [17] analyzed the predictive value of abnormal MRI features for the survival of patients with GBM. The result demonstrated that tumor burden and invasion characteristics indicated by the T1-weighted gadolinium-enhanced MRI were significant predictors of patient survival, but the total area of signal intensity abnormalities on the T2-weighted images and the T2/T1 ratio did not correlate with patient outcome.

In summary, for patients with GBM, the significance of peritumoral edema for the survival of a patient with GBM is not clear. A majority of tumor tissues are contained within the contrast enhancement areas in T1-weighted MRI, but not always, and infiltrate into the peritumoral edema area. We believe that GTV in HGG for RT should be focus in T1-weighted MRI and surgical bed, regarding the peritumoral edema area. In addition, the ability to accurately distinguish tumor-infiltrated edema from vasogenic edema composed purely of extracellular water could be helpful for target delineation. It is hoped that advances in image techniques will enable this in the future.

2.2 Recurrent patterns of postoperative GBM

Several studies have studied the pattern of relapse in patients with glioblastoma. One of them [18] retrospectively analyzed the patterns of radiographic presentation of 80 adult patients with supratentorial GBM at four clinically relevant time points: presentation, first recurrence, second recurrence, and third recurrence. At diagnosis, 87.5% (70/80), 6.25% (5/80), 3.75%, and 2.5% of patients presented with unifocal disease and distant, multifocal, and diffuse MRI-defined radiographic patterns, respectively. After RT and temozolamide treatment local recurrence occurs in 80%, distant in 7,5% and multifocal in 6,25% (including one with cerebrospinal fluid dissemination), and 6.25% was diffuse. In the same way, Wallner et al. [19] found that 78% of unifocal anaplastic astrocytoma and GBM recurrences occurred within 2 cm of the presurgical original tumor extent, which is defined as the enhancing edge of the tumor on preoperative CT, and 56% (18/32) of tumors recurred within 1 cm of the initial tumor margin. Liang et al. [20] published the pattern of failure for 42 patients with grade III or IV astrocytoma treated with chemoradiotherapy to a total of 60 Gy. In all 42 patients, recurrence occurred within a 2 cm margin of the original CT-enhancing lesion, and 10% of the patients suffered from multifocal recurrence. In a retrospective series of 34 patients treated either with WBRT and conformal boost or entirely with 3D conformal RT, Oppitz et al. [21] revealed that all GBM recurrences occurred within the 90% isodose line when targets were contoured around the original preoperative contrast-enhancing tumor plus a 2 cm margin. More than 80% of the recurrences occur in 2 cm of the surgical bed dose-escalation studies analyzed 36 patients with HGGs treated with radiation alone to 70–80 Gy using the 3D conformal techniques [22]. In this study, recurrences were divided into several categories: (1) "central," in which 95% or more of the recurrent tumor volume (Vrecur) was within D95, the region treated to a high dose (95% of the prescription dose); (2) "infield," in which 80% or more of V recur was within the D95 isodose surface; (3) "marginal," when between 20 and 80% of Vrecur was inside the D95 surface; and (4) "outwith," in which <20% of Vrecur was inside the D95 surface. This study found that 89% of the recurrences were central or infield, 3/36 (8%) had a marginal recurrence pattern, and only one patient (3%) clearly failed outside of the high-dose region. Another trial [7] reported similar patterns of failure in a series of 48 patients with GBM, comparing treatment guidelines based on residual tumor and cavity plus 2 cm margin, as used at the MD Anderson Cancer Center, with RTOG guidelines that specified the inclusion of preoperative peritumoral edema. They showed that 90% (43/48) of patients failed in central and infield locations. The five remaining marginal and distal recurrences failed to be covered by the 46 Gy isodose line, even when overlaid by the RTOG plan incorporating edema volume, confirming them to be true marginal recurrences. Additionally, Minniti et al. [23] compared recurrence patterns in 105 patients whose surgical resections were delineated by the EORTC contouring technique, wherein the CTV includes the resection cavity, and any residual tumor seen on postoperative T1-weighted MRI, plus a 2 cm margin, and the PTV includes the CTV plus an additional 3 mm margin. After recurrence was confirmed, a theoretical plan, based on the addition of postoperative edema plus 2 cm margins, according to the current

RTOG guidelines, was created for each patient. The radiation coverage of the site of subsequent recurrences was compared for the different contouring techniques. The results revealed no significant differences in relapse patterns between the two target delineation techniques. Although, the median percent volume of normal brain irradiated to high doses was significantly smaller using the EORTC guideline. In our opinion, these data provide some evidence and reassurance to support treatment plans based on resection cavity and any residual tumor seen on postoperative T1-weighted MRI with a 2 cm margin, rather than specified inclusion of preoperative peritumoral edema plus a 2 cm margin. The use of this limited-margin RT can significantly decrease the volume of normal brain tissue that is irradiated, without a significant increase in the risk of marginal recurrences. A number of studies have been conducted to explore the feasibility of limited-margin RT in the context of a treatment paradigm involving RT with concurrent chemotherapy. Trying to reduce treatment volume, McDonald et al. [8] report the pattern of tumor failure in a series of 62 patients with GBM treated with postoperative limited-margin RT and concurrent chemotherapy. The initial CTV included the postoperative T2 abnormality, with a median margin of 0.7 cm. The boost CTV included the residual T1-enhancing tumor and resection cavity, with a median margin of 0.5 cm. The PTV margin varied from an additional 0.3 cm–0.5 cm. The initial dose was 46–54 Gy, followed by a boost to 60 Gy. In this study, the total boost PTV (PTV_{boost}) margin was 1 cm or less in 92% of the patients. Results showed that 38/41 patients (93%) had a central or infield failure, two (5%) had a marginal failure, and one (2%) had a distant failure, relative to the 60 Gy isodose line. The author concluded that a PTV_{boost} margin of 1 cm or less did not appear to increase the risk of marginal and/or distant tumor failure, compared with other published series. In the same direction, Dobelbower et al. [24] analyzed the patterns of failure in patients with GBM treated with concurrent radiation and TMZ. Patients generally received 46 Gy to the primary tumor, surrounding edema, plus a 1 cm margin and 60 Gy to the enhancing tumor plus a 1 cm margin. The result revealed that 18 patients (90%) had infield failures, 2 patients (10%) had marginal failures, and no regional failures were reported. Four patients (20%) suffered from distant failure, in which an independent satellite lesion was located completely outwith the 95% isodose curve. These studies also suggested that by delineating the GTV based on peritumoral edema, it is feasible to reduce the margin to 1 cm or less. Clinical studies showed that the volume of irradiated brain is important factor in the development of neurotoxicity and for the development of radiographic and pathologic surrogates for neurotoxicity [25–28].

Smaller RT fields may be more appropriate than larger RT fields, possibly reducing the risk of late neurological deterioration especially in patients with large peritumoral edema. The neurocognitive function would be likely to be affected by radiation therapy especially in long-term survivors [29].

The pattern of failure for GBM after radiation therapy has been studied previously; almost all tumors fail within a 2 cm margin of the resection cavity or residual tumor. The primary failure location was infield, but some patients had marginal failures, and few had a distant failure or an independent satellite lesion. Taking these data into consideration, we conclude that it is preferable to contour the GTV based on the T1-enhanced MRI, and regard the peritumoral edema as a subclinical lesion. We suggest that the CTV should be identified based on the residual T1-enhancing tumor and resection cavity (GTV) with a 2 cm margin or the postoperative T2 or FLAIR (fluid-attenuated inversion recovery) abnormality; however, in the case of a cone-down boost phase, the CTV should include the GTV with a 1 cm margin.

3. Dose

Standard therapy for HGG patients is a total dose of 60 Gy in 30–33 fractions [30]. Adequate doses of RT are required to maximize the survival benefit [31–33]. One important study conducted by Walker et al. evaluated the relationship between survival and increasing doses of RT in malign gliomas [33]. Doses ranged from <45 Gy to 60 Gy. They showed that there was a significant improvement in median survival from 28 to 42 weeks in the groups treated with doses of 50–60 Gy. There is no benefit for dose escalation of >60 Gy. In two randomized trials, there were no significant differences in tumor control or survival in patients treated with 60 Gy cranial radiation or 60 Gy followed by a 10 Gy tumor boost [34, 35]. Two series [35, 36] analyzed failure patterns for patients with HGG dose escalation levels 70, 80, and 90 Gy. The GTV was defined based on postoperative gadolinium-enhanced T1-weighted images. They defined three separate PTVs in three dimensions by 0.5 cm to make PTV1, 1.5 cm to make PTV2, and 2.5 cm to make PTV3 from GTV. At median follow-up of 11.7 months, median survival was found to be 11.7 months, and 1- and 2-year survivals were 47.1% and 12.9%, respectively. The authors concluded that despite dose escalation to 90 Gy, the predominant failure pattern in HGG remained local. This suggested that close margins used in highly conformal treatments did not increase the risk of marginal or distant recurrences. Since the majority of tumor recurrences were seen within the previous radiation therapy fields and the poor outcomes associated with standard regimen, the new therapy strategies were evaluated to deliver higher doses to the tumor bed. Higher doses for HGG have been attempted with a variety of methods, including altered fractionation [37, 38], stereotactic radio surgery [39], and brachytherapy [40].

The term "conventional RT" refers to giving daily radiation of 180–200 cGy per day. "Hypofractionated RT" refers to the use of a higher daily dose of radiation (> 200 cGy per day) which typically reduces the overall number of fractions and therefore the overall treatment time. "Hyperfractionated RT" defined as the use of a lower daily dose of radiation (< 180 cGy per day), a greater number of fractions and multiple fractions delivered per day in order to deliver a total dose at least equivalent to external beam daily conventionally fractionated RT in the same time frame. The aim of this approach is to reduce the potential for late toxicity [41, 42]. In this study, the authors compared hyperfractionated RT (with or without chemotherapy) vs. conventionally fractionated RT (without chemotherapy). The trial included 81 HGG patients randomized to conventional fractionation (5800 cGy in 30 daily fractions) or hyperfractionation (6141 cGy in 89 cGy fractions given 3 times a day every 2–4 hours for 4.5 weeks). Median survival in two groups was 39 and 27 weeks, respectively, and the 1-year survival rates were 41 and 20%, respectively. Others have failed to confirm these results. Therefore, there is insufficient data regarding hyperfractionation vs. conventionally fractionated radiation (without chemotherapy) and insufficient data regarding accelerated radiation vs. conventionally fractionated radiation (without chemotherapy) [43].

"Hypofractionated RT" refers to the delivery of higher daily dose to reduce the overall treatment time. Five studies that randomized participants to hypofractionated radiation therapy vs. conventionally fractionated RT [43]. Their results suggested that hypofractionated RT has similar efficacy for survival as compared to conventional radiotherapy, especially for individuals aged 60 and older with HGG. A randomized controlled trial (RCT) and several retrospective studies conducted in the elderly suggest that short course-radiation therapy (SCRT) of 34–40 Gy in 2.6–3.4 Gy fractions, with or without TMZ, may have similar results to LCRT [44–46]. Results from the Nordic trial suggested that SCRT may be superior to LCRT in patients aged ≥70 years [47]. An International Atomic Energy Agency Randomized Phase III Study of Radiation Therapy in Elderly and/or Frail Patients with Newly Diagnosed Glioblastoma Multiforme showed no differences in overall survival time, progression-free survival time, and quality of life between patients receiving the two radiotherapy regimens (25 Gy in five daily fractions over 1 week vs. 40 Gy in 15 daily fractions over 3 weeks) [48].

There are no data comparing optimal dose and schedule in grade III gliomas vs. GBM. However, many radiation oncologists use a dose of 59.4 Gy in 1.8 Gy fractions for grade III tumors vs. 60 Gy in 2 Gy fractions for grade IV tumors with the expectation that dose reduction per fraction may lead to reduced late normal tissue effects for patients with probability longer-term survival [49].

4. Stereotactic radiotherapy and radiosurgery (SRS)

Stereotactic radiotherapy or radiosurgery (SRS) uses three-dimensional planning techniques to precisely deliver narrowly collimated beams of ionizing radiation in a single high-dose fraction to small lesions [50, 51]. This technique in primary treatment of HGG was used in some trials a boost (additional dose). The treatment was composed of 50 Gy conventional RT and four SRT boost fractions of either 5 or 7 Gy. SRT was administered once weekly during the final 4 weeks of therapy. The results suggested that while the regimen was safe, there was no survival benefit compared to the standard of care. Some retrospective studies suggest that it may be used in patients with recurrent HGG previously irradiated. A number of small prospective and retrospective series suggest that SRS may prolong survival in this setting, either alone or in combination with chemotherapy [52]. It is important to know the bias of these studies including the initial radiation dose, extent of initial and second surgical resections, tumor volume at the time of SRS, and timing and use of chemotherapy and the time between initial radiation therapy and retreatment have clear implications on patient outcomes but are variably reported [52, 53]. Patients newly diagnosed with progressive/recurrent gliomas, there is insufficient evidence in terms of the benefits/harms of using SRS/SRT. There is also insufficient evidence regarding the benefits/harms in the use of SRS/SRT at the time of progression or recurrence.

5. Reirradiation in recurrent high-grade gliomas

Tumor recurrence is inevitable in HGG patients, but diagnostic of progressive disease from radiation necrosis or other radiation-induced imaging changes could be a big challenge. Treatment decisions for patients with recurrent or progressive HGG must be individualized, since therapy is not curative and there are no randomized trials that directly compare active intervention vs. supportive care. Reoperation is an important treatment modality and may involve either biopsy (for diagnostic purposes) or repeat debulking of tumor, but only 20–30% of recurrent HGG patients are candidates for another surgery [54]. Focal RT approaches are often employed with limited volume recurrences; however, the role of reirradiation in patients with recurrent HGG is uncertain, and there is a lack of prospective data. Based on retrospective series, selected patients with small recurrent tumors and a good performance status may benefit from repeat radiation using modern high-precision techniques [55]. In a small series of 101 patients with recurrent HGG, the median survival was 12 months for patients with grade III tumors and 8 months for those with grade IV lesions. In this study SBRT was performed with a median dose of 36 Gy (range 15–62) [56].

6. Toxicity of radiotherapy

The toxicity of RT usually divided into acute and late effects, effects differentiated by time that occur, during radiation or up to 3 months afterward, early-delayed effects that appear up to 6 months after radiation, and late effects that can develop 6 months or more after the completion of radiation. Usually, acute reactions are reversible, and late reactions are generally irreversible. Most common acute radiation morbidity during cranial irradiation includes fatigue, erythema, alopecia, headache, and nausea with or without vomiting; these are usually not severe and are self-limiting [49]. The factors influencing the likelihood of developing complications include the volume of normal brain tissue treated and the total radiation dose. Fatigue is one of the most common side effects of cranial irradiation. In a prospective study with 70 consecutive patients receiving radical cranial irradiation, most of the patients were treated for GBM, and their results suggested that 90% of the patients experienced ≥ grade 1 symptoms (disturbance with some tiredness, but activity not curtailed), and approximately half experienced mild to moderate symptoms like decreased activity and increased tiredness, sleeping much of the day or most activities curtailed. The symptoms typically began within 2 weeks of the start of RT, peaked at approximately 6–8 weeks, and then slowly resolved over the next several months. Corticosteroids or antiemetic are used to prevent or abbreviate the symptoms. Late effects including cognitive impairments and radiation necrosis are worrisome and may become manifest many years after RT [57]. Cranial irradiation can result in a spectrum of neurocognitive deficits in the years following treatment in children and in adults. The data of radiation-induced cognitive impairment is mostly learned from studies that are conducted in low-grade glioma patients. Cognitive functioning in patients with brain tumor was affected by the antiepileptic drug use, extent of surgery, tumor localization, and age [57]. Radiation necrosis is a serious and uncommon late toxicity that typically develops 1–3 years after radiation, but in rare cases it has been reported more than 10 years after radiation [58]. The probability of radiation necrosis is strict dependence on the dose. Focal brain radiation with doses around 70 Gy using conventional 2 Gy fractionation risk of focal radiation necrosis is usually estimated in 5% in 5 years [59]. The risk of radiation necrosis probably increases with concurrent chemotherapy or radio sensitizers [60].

7. Conclusion

The standard of care for HGG adults, up to age 70 with good performance status, is conformal fractionated radiotherapy (6000 cGy in 30 daily fractions) with the addition of concurrent and adjuvant temozolomide chemotherapy following maximal safe debulking of the tumor. Elderly patients, older than 70 years or with poor performance status, hypofractionated RT has similar efficacy for survival as compared to conventional radiotherapy.

The optimal treatment volume for HGG patients remains controversial and varies among cooperative groups; dose escalation above 60 Gy or stereotactic radiosurgery has not shown any survival benefits. Treatment decisions for patients with recurrent or progressive HGG must be individualized, since therapy is not curative and there are no randomized trials that directly compare active intervention vs. supportive care.

Author details

Henrique Balloni
Department of Radiation Oncology of Oncoville Oncoville, Curitiba PR, Brazil

*Address all correspondence to: henriqueballoni@gmail.com

IntechOpen

© 2019 The Author(s). Licensee IntechOpen. This chapter is distributed under the terms of the Creative Commons Attribution License (http://creativecommons.org/licenses/by/3.0), which permits unrestricted use, distribution, and reproduction in any medium, provided the original work is properly cited.

References

[1] Stupp R, Mason WP, van den Bent MJ, et al. Radiotherapy plus concomitant and adjuvant temozolomide for glioblastoma. The New England Journal of Medicine. 2005;**352**(10):987-996. DOI: 10.1056/NEJMoa043330

[2] Walker MD, Alexander E Jr, Hunt WE, et al. Evaluation of BCNU and/or radiotherapy in the treatment of anaplastic gliomas. A cooperative clinical trial. Journal of Neurosurgery. 1978;**49**(3):333-343. DOI: 10.3171/jns.1978.49.3.0333

[3] Shapiro WR, Green SB, Burger PC, et al. Randomized trial of three chemotherapy regimens and two radiotherapy regimens and two radiotherapy regimens in postoperative treatment of malignant glioma. Brain tumor cooperative group trial 8001. Journal of Neurosurgery. 1989;**71**(1):1-9. DOI: 10.3171/jns.1989.71.1.0001

[4] Heesters MA, Wijrdeman HK, Struikmans H, Witkamp T, Moerland MA. Brain tumor delineation based on CT and MR imaging. Implications for radiotherapy treatment planning. Strahlentherapie und Onkologie. 1993;**169**(12):729-733. PMI 8284745

[5] Leibel SA, Scott CB, Loeffler JS. Contemporary approaches to the treatment of malignant gliomas with radiation therapy. Seminars in Oncology. 1994;**21**(2):198-219. PMID: 8153665

[6] Colman H, Berkey BA, Maor MH, et al. Phase II radiation therapy oncology group trial of conventional radiation therapy followed by treatment with recombinant interferon-beta for supratentorial glioblastoma: Results of RTOG 9710. International Journal of Radiation Oncology, Biology, Physics. 2006;**66**(3):818-824. DOI: 10.1016/j.ijrobp.2006.05.021

[7] Chang EL, Akyurek S, Avalos T, et al. Evaluation of peritumoral edema in the delineation of radiotherapy clinical target volumes for glioblastoma. International Journal of Radiation Oncology, Biology, Physics. 2007;**68**(1):144-150. DOI: 10.1016/j.ijrobp.2006.12.009

[8] McDonald MW, Shu HK, Curran WJ Jr, Crocker IR. Pattern of failure after limited margin radiotherapy and temozolomide for glioblastoma. International Journal of Radiation Oncology, Biology, Physics. 2011;**79**(1):130-136. DOI: 10.1016/j.ijrobp.2009.10.048

[9] Ghose A, Lim G, Husain S. Treatment for glioblastoma multiforme: Current guidelines and Canadian practice. Current Oncology. 2010;**17**(6):52-58. PMID: 21151410

[10] Burger PC, Dubois PJ, Schold SC Jr, et al. Computerized tomographic and pathologic studies of the untreated, quiescent, and recurrent glioblastoma multiforme. Journal of Neurosurgery. 1983;**58**(2):159-169. DOI: 10.3171/jns.1983.58.2.0159

[11] Halperin EC, Bentel G, Heinz ER, Burger PC. Radiation therapy treatment planning in supratentorial glioblastoma multiforme: An analysis based on post mortem topographic anatomy with CT correlations. International Journal of Radiation Oncology, Biology, Physics. 1989;**17**(6):1347-1350. PMID:2557310

[12] Kelly PJ, Daumas-Duport C, Kispert DB, Kall BA, Scheithauer BW, Illig JJ. Imaging-based stereotaxic serial biopsies in untreated intracranial glial neoplasms. Journal of Neurosurgery. 1987;**66**(6):865-874. DOI: 10.3171/jns.1987.66.6.0865

[13] Lu S, Ahn D, Johnson G, Law M, Zagzag D, Grossman

RI. Diffusion-tensor MR imaging of intracranial neoplasia and associated peritumoral edema: Introduction of the tumor infiltration index. Radiology. 2004;**232**(1):221-228. DOI: 10.1148/radiol.2321030653

[14] Schoenegger K, Oberndorfer S, Wuschitz B, et al. Peritumoral edema on MRI at initial diagnosis: An independent prognostic factor for glioblastoma? European Journal of Neurology. 2009;**16**(7):874-878. DOI: 10.3171/jns.1987.66.6.0865

[15] Pope WB, Sayre J, Perlina A, Villablanca JP, Mischel PS, Cloughesy TF. MR imaging correlates of survival in patients with high-grade gliomas. AJNR. American Journal of Neuroradiology. 2005;**26**(10): 2466-2474. PMID:16286386

[16] Iliadis G, Kotoula V, Chatzisotiriou A, et al. Volumetric and MGMT parameters in glioblastoma patients: Survival analysis. BMC Cancer. 2012;**12**:3. DOI: 10.1186/1471-2407-12-3

[17] Ramakrishna R, Barber J, Kennedy G, et al. Imaging features of invasion and preoperative and postoperative tumor burden in previously untreated glioblastoma: Correlation with survival. Surgical Neurology International. 2010;**1**:40. DOI: 10.4103/2152-7806.68337

[18] Chamberlain MC. Radiographic patterns of relapse in glioblastoma. Journal of Neuro-Oncology. 2011;**101**(2):319-323. DOI: 10.1007/s11060-010-0251-4

[19] Wallner KE, Galicich JH, Krol G, Arbit E, Malkin MG. Patterns of failure following treatment for glioblastoma multiforme and anaplastic astrocytoma. International Journal of Radiation Oncology, Biology, Physics. 1989;**16**(6):1405-1409. PMID:2542195

[20] Liang BC, Thornton AF Jr, Sandler HM, Greenberg HS. Malignant astrocytomas: Focal tumor recurrence after focal external beam radiation therapy. Journal of Neurosurgery. 1991;**75**(4):559-563. DOI: 10.3171/jns.1991.75.4.0559

[21] Oppitz U, Maessen D, Zunterer H, Richter S, Flentje M. 3D-recurrence-patterns of glioblastomas after CT-planned postoperative irradiation. Radiotherapy and Oncology. 1999;**53**(1):53-57. DOI: 10.1186/s13014-016-0665-z

[22] Lee SW, Fraass BA, Marsh LH, et al. Patterns of failure following high-dose 3-D conformal radiotherapy for high-grade astrocytomas: A quantitative dosimetric study. International Journal of Radiation Oncology, Biology, Physics. 1999;**43**(1):79-88. PMID:9989517

[23] Minniti G, Amelio D, Amichetti M, et al. Patterns of failure and comparison of different target volume delineations in patients with glioblastoma treated with conformal radiotherapy plus concomitant and adjuvant temozolomide. Radiotherapy and Oncology. 2010;**97**(3):377-381. DOI: 10.1016/j.radonc.2010.08.020

[24] Dobelbower MC, Burnett Iii OL, Nordal RA, et al. Patterns of failure for glioblastoma multiforme following concurrent radiation and temozolomide. Journal of Medical Imaging and Radiation Oncology. 2011;**55**(1):77-81. DOI: 10.1111/j.1754-9485.2010.02232.x

[25] Klein M, Heimans JJ, Aaronson NK, et al. Effect of radiotherapy and other treatment-related factors on mid-term to long-term cognitive sequelae in low-grade gliomas: A comparative study. Lancet. 2002;**360**(9343):1361-1368. PMID:12423981

[26] Kleinberg L, Wallner K, Malkin MG. Good performance status of

long-term disease-free survivors of intracranial gliomas. International Journal of Radiation Oncology, Biology, Physics. 1993;**26**(1):129-133. DOI: 10.1016/0360-3016(93)90183-V

[27] Marks JE, Baglan RJ, Prassad SC, Blank WF. Cerebral radionecrosis: Incidence and risk in relation to dose, time, fractionation and volume. International Journal of Radiation Oncology, Biology, Physics. 1981;7(2):243-252. PMC1014206

[28] Swennen MH, Bromberg JE, Witkamp TD, Terhaard CH, Postma TJ, Taphoorn MJ. Delayed radiation toxicity after focal or whole brain radiotherapy for low-grade glioma. Journal of Neuro-Oncology. 2004;**66**(3):333-339. DOI: 10.1120/jacmp.v8i2.2423

[29] Jalali R, Mallick I, Dutta D, et al. Factors influencing neurocognitive outcomes in young patients with benign and low-grade brain tumors treated with stereotactic conformal radiotherapy. International Journal of Radiation Oncology, Biology, Physics. 2010;**77**(4):974-979. DOI: 10.1016/j.ijrobp.2009.06.025

[30] Gondi V, Pugh SL, Tome WA, Caine C, Corn B, Kanner A, et al. Preservation of memory with conformal avoidance of the hippocampal neural stem-cell compartment during whole-brain radiotherapy for brain metastases (RTOG 0933): A phase II multi-institutional trial. Journal of Clinical Oncology. 2014;**32**:3810-3816

[31] Kirkpatrick JP, Laack NN, Shih HA, Gondi V. Management of GBM: A problem of local recurrence. Adjuvant Radiation Therapy for High-Grade Gliomas. Journal of Neuro-Oncology; 2017

[32] Coffey RJ, Lunsford LD, Taylor FH. Survival after stereotactic biopsy of malignant gliomas. Neurosurgery. 1988;**22**:465-473

[33] Walker MD, Strike TA, Sheline GE. An analysis of dose-effect relationship in the radiotherapy of malignant gliomas. International Journal of Radiation Oncology, Biology, Physics. 1979;**5**:1725-1731

[34] Nelson DF, Diener-West M, Horton J, Chang CH, Schoenfeld D, Nelson JS. Combined modality approach to treatment of malignant gliomas--re-evaluation of RTOG 7401/ECOG 1374 with long-term follow-up: A joint study of the radiation therapy oncology group and the eastern cooperative oncology group. NCI Monographs. 1988:279-284

[35] Lee SW, Fraass BA, Marsh LH, Herbort K, Gebarski SS, Martel MK, et al. Patterns of failure following high-dose 3-D conformal radiotherapy for high-grade astrocytomas: A quantitative dosimetric study. International Journal of Radiation Oncology, Biology, Physics. 1999;**43**:79-88

[36] Chan JL, Lee SW, Fraass BA, Normolle DP, Greenberg HS, Junck LR, et al. Survival and failure patterns of high-grade gliomas after three-dimensional conformal radiotherapy. Journal of Clinical Oncology. 2002;**20**:1635-1642

[37] Werner-Wasik M, Scott CB, Nelson DF, Gaspar LE, Murray KJ, Fischbach JA, et al. Final report of a phase I/II trial of hyperfractionated and accelerated hyperfractionated radiation therapy with carmustine for adults with supratentorial malignant gliomas: Radiation therapy oncology group study 83-02. Cancer. 1996;**77**:1535-1543

[38] Nieder C, Nestle U, Ketter R, Kolles H, Gentner SJ, Steudel WI, et al. Hyperfractionated and accelerated-hyperfractionated radiotherapy for glioblastoma multiforme. Radiation Oncology Investigations. 1999;**7**:36-41

[39] Mehta MP, Masciopinto J, Rozental J, Levin A, Chappell R, Bastin K, et al. Stereotactic radiosurgery for glioblastoma multiforme: Report of a prospective study evaluating prognostic factors and analyzing long-term survival advantage. International Journal of Radiation Oncology. 1994;**30**:541-549

[40] Sneed PK, Lamborn KR, Larson DA, Prados MD, Malec MK, McDermott MW, et al. Demonstration of brachytherapy boost dose-response relationships in glioblastoma multiforme. International Journal of Radiation Oncology, Biology, Physics. 1996;**35**:37-44

[41] Shin KH, Muller PJ, Geggie PH. Superfractionation radiation therapy in the treatment of malignant astrocytoma. Cancer. 1983;**52**:2040-2043

[42] Lorentini S, Amelio D, Giri MG, Fellin F, Meliado G, Rizzotti A, et al. IMRT or 3D-CRT in glioblastoma? A dosimetric criterion for patient selection. Technology in Cancer Research & Treatment. 2013;**12**:411-420

[43] Khan L, Soliman H, Sahgal A, Perry J, Xu W, Tsao MN. External beam radiation dose escalation for high grade glioma. Cochrane Database of Systematic Reviews. 2016;**8**:011475

[44] Roa W, Brasher PM, Bauman G, Anthes M, Bruera E, Chan A, et al. Abbreviated course of radiation therapy in older patients with glioblastoma multiforme: A prospective randomized clinical trial. Journal of Clinical Oncology. 2004;**22**:1583-1588

[45] Arvold ND, Tanguturi SK, Aizer AA, Wen PY, Reardon DA, Lee EQ, et al. Hypofractionated versus standard radiation therapy with or without temozolomide for older glioblastoma patients. International Journal of Radiation Oncology, Biology, Physics. 2015;**92**:384-389

[46] Minniti G, De Sanctis V, Muni R, Rasio D, Lanzetta G, Bozzao A, et al. Hypofractionated radiotherapy followed by adjuvant chemotherapy with temozolomide in elderly patients with glioblastoma. Journal of Neuro-Oncology. 2009;**91**:95-100

[47] Malmstrom A, Gronberg BH, Marosi C, Stupp R, Frappaz D, Schultz H, et al. Temozolomide versus standard 6-week radiotherapy versus hypofractionated radiotherapy in patients older than 60 years with glioblastoma: The Nordic randomised, phase 3 trial. The Lancet Oncology. 2012;**13**:916-926

[48] Roa W, Kepka L, Kumar N, Sinaika V, et al. International Atomic Energy Agency randomized phase III study of radiation therapy in elderly and/or frail patients with newly diagnosed glioblastoma multiforme. Journal of Clinical Oncology. 2015;**33**(35):4145-4150. DOI: 10.1200/JCO.2015.62.6606

[49] Lassman AB, Matceyevsky D, Corn BW. High-grade gliomas. In: Clinical Radiation Oncology. 4th ed. USA: Elsevier; 2016

[50] Ten Haken RK, Thornton AF, Sandler HM, LaVigne ML, Quint DJ, Fraass BA, et al. A quantitative assessment of the addition of MRI to CT-based, 3-D treatment planning of brain tumors. Radiotherapy and Oncology. 1992;**25**:121-133

[51] Douglas JG, Stelzer KJ, Mankoff DA, Tralins KS, Krohn KA, Muzi M, et al. [F-18]-fluorodeoxyglucose positron emission tomography for targeting radiation dose escalation for patients with glioblastoma multiforme: Clinical outcomes and patterns of failure. International Journal of Radiation Oncology. 2006;**64**:886

[52] Redmond KJ, Mehta M. Stereotactic radiosurgery for glioblastoma. Cureus. 2015;7(12):e413

[53] Murovic JA, Chang SD. Outcomes after stereotactic radiosurgery and various adjuvant treatments for recurrent glioblastoma multiforme: A current literature review and comparison of multiple factors that impact outcome. World Neurosurgery. 2012;**78**:588-591

[54] Weller M, van den Bent M, Tonn JC, Stupp R, Preusser M, CohenJonathan-Moyal E, et al. European Association for Neuro-Oncology(EANO) guideline on the diagnosis and treatment of adult astrocytic and oligodendroglial gliomas. The Lancet Oncology. 2017;**18**:315

[55] National Comprehensive Cancer Network (NCCN). NCCN Clinical Practice Guidelines in Oncology

[56] Combs SE, Thilmann C, Edler L, Debus J, Schulz-Ertner D. Efficacy of fractionated stereotactic reirradiation in recurrent gliomas: Long-term results in 172 patients treated in a single institution. Journal of Clinical Oncology. 2005;**23**:8863-8869

[57] Douw L, Klein M, Fagel SS, Van den Heuvel J, Taphoorn MJ, Aaronson NK, et al. Cognitive and radiological effects of radiotherapy in patients with low-grade glioma: Long-term follow-up. Lancet Neurology. 2009;**8**(9):810-818

[58] Strenger V, Lackner H, Mayer R, Sminia P, Sovinz P, Mokry M, et al. Incidence and clinical course of radionecrosis in children with brain tumors. A 20-year longitudinal observational study. Strahlentherapie und Onkologie. 2013;**189**:759-764

[59] Leibel S, Sheline G. Tolerance of the brain and spinal cord to conventional therapeutic irradiation. In: Gutin P, Leibel S, Sheline G, editors. Radiation Injury to the Nervous System. Raven Press; 1991. p. 239

[60] Ruben JD, Dally M, Bailey M, Smith R, Mc Lean CA, Fedele P. Cerebral radiation necrosis: Incidence, outcomes, and risk factors with emphasis on radiation parameters and chemotherapy. International Journal of Radiation Oncology, Biology, Physics. 2006;**65**:499-508